A Pest in the Land

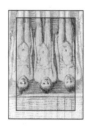

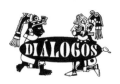

Diálogos Series

KRIS LANE, SERIES EDITOR

Understanding Latin America demands dialogue, deep exploration, and frank discussion of key topics. Founded by Lyman L. Johnson in 1992 and edited since 2013 by Kris Lane, the Diálogos Series focuses on innovative scholarship in Latin American history and related fields. The series, the most successful of its type, includes specialist works accessible to a wide readership and a variety of thematic titles, all ideally suited for classroom adoption by university and college teachers.

Also available in the Diálogos Series:

Creating Charismatic Bonds in Argentina by Donna Guy
Gendered Crossings: Women and Migration in the Spanish Empire
by Allyson M. Poska
From Shipmates to Soldiers: Emerging Black Identities in the Río de la Plata
by Alex Borucki
Women Drug Traffickers: Mules, Bosses, and Organized Crime by Elaine Carey
Searching for Madre Matiana: Prophecy and Popular Culture in Modern Mexico
by Edward Wright-Rios
Africans into Creoles: Slavery, Ethnicity, and Identity in Colonial Costa Rica
by Russell Lohse
Native Brazil: Beyond the Convert and the Cannibal, 1500–1900
edited by Hal Langfur
Emotions and Daily Life in Colonial Mexico
edited by Javier Villa-Flores and Sonya Lipsett-Rivera
The Course of Andean History by Peter V. N. Henderson
Masculinity and Sexuality in Modern Mexico
edited by Anne Rubenstein and Víctor M. Macías-González

For additional titles in the Diálogos Series, please visit unmpress.com.

A Pest in the Land

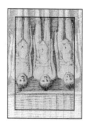

NEW WORLD EPIDEMICS IN A GLOBAL PERSPECTIVE

Suzanne Austin Alchon

UNIVERSITY OF NEW MEXICO PRESS

ALBUQUERQUE

For my parents,
Hadley Warner Austin and Elizabeth Coombs Austin,
and my daughter,
Lilla Aimée Austin Alchon

© 2003 by the University of New Mexico Press
All rights reserved.
Printed in the United States of America
21 20 19 18 17 16   2 3 4 5 6 7
Paperbound ISBN-13: 978-0-8263-2871-7

Library of Congress Cataloging-in-Publication Data

Alchon, Suzanne Austin.
A pest in the land : new world epidemics in a global perspective /
Suzanne Austin Alchon.— 1st ed.
p. cm. — (Dialogos series)
Includes bibliographical references and index.
ISBN 0-8263-2870-9 (cloth : alk. paper) —
ISBN 0-8263-2871-7 (pbk. : alk. paper)
1. Medical geography—Latin America.   2. Epidemiology—Latin America.
3. Communicable diseases—Latin America—History.   I. Title.
II. Series: Dialogos (Albuquerque, N.M.)
RA792.A436 2002
614.4′2′098—dc21
2002151378

Design: Melissa Tandysh

• Contents •

• *List of Illustrations* •

Tables

• *Acknowledgments* •

The idea for this book originated with Professor Lyman Johnson, fellow Latin American historian and series advisory editor for Diálogos. Throughout the process of conceptualizing and writing, Lyman has been unfailing in his encouragement, insightful in his suggestions, thorough in his editing, and generous in his praise. In addition, I am also indebted to David Holtby, editor in chief of the University of New Mexico Press, for his ongoing support of this project. The staff of the Morris Library of the University of Delaware, and in particular those individuals in the interlibrary loan office, deserve special praise for helping me track down many an obscure reference. In addition, I wish to thank Shelly McCoy for sharing her invaluable knowledge of mapping technology. Special thanks also go to my friend and colleague Professor Ray Nichols, who came to the rescue when I was faced with what seemed to me the insurmountable task of digitizing the images used in this book. Most recently, Karen Taschek has been both patient and thorough in copyediting the manuscript. Finally, I want to thank Thomas M. DiLorenzo, colleague and friend, for his enthusiastic support of this project.

• Introduction •

We always want to believe that history happened only to "them," "in the past," and that somehow we are outside history, rather than enmeshed within it. Many aspects of history are unanticipated and unforeseen, predictable only in retrospect. . . . Yet in one vital area, the emergence and spread of new infectious diseases, we can already predict the future—and it is threatening and dangerous to us all. . . . The history of our time will be marked by recurrent eruptions of newly discovered diseases.

Laurie Garrett, *The Coming Plague*

Many of us who live in the United States at the beginning of the twenty-first century often forget that we remain as vulnerable to the emergence and spread of new infectious diseases as all other human populations, past and present. That we have lost sight of this central fact of human existence reveals much about our misplaced confidence in the medical profession and our seemingly boundless optimism regarding the development of medical technologies and drug therapies. But in her book *The Coming Plague*, medical writer Laurie Garrett argues persuasively that our confidence and optimism are sheer hubris and that, in fact, modern technologies and the rapid worldwide movement of people only facilitate the transfer of diseases from one region to another and increase the likelihood of the appearance of new infectious illnesses. One has only to look at the recent outbreaks of Bolivian hemorrhagic fever, Lassa fever, Ebola, and acquired immune deficiency syndrome (AIDS) to realize that the evolutionary relationship between humans and disease-causing organisms continues unabated.

In addition to these new threats, even as the twenty-first century begins, a host of infectious diseases long known to human populations continues to exact a heavy toll: in 1993 measles infected 45 million worldwide, killing 1.2 million children. That same year, the World Health Organization reported 600,000 new cases of leprosy. All told, in 1993, communicable diseases, most of them with centuries-long histories among human communities, claimed the lives of some 20 million individuals around the world. While the vast majority of these deaths occurred in Asia, Africa, the Middle East, and Latin America—that is, among the poor of the so-called developing world—to those of us living in the industrialized nations of the West, these statistics are yet another powerful reminder that our complaisance is at best misplaced.

Since ours is but the most recent chapter in the ongoing history of humans and infectious disease, it is instructive to look back at other periods when the relationship between people and pathogens was particularly volatile. For such an example, one need look no farther than "the Age of European Exploration," when, beginning in the fifteenth century, Portuguese voyages along the African coast inaugurated a period of global exploration and massive human migrations, both forced and voluntary, that has only accelerated until the present time. This is a book about the timeless and universal nature of the human experience with disease. It argues that all human populations respond to their initial encounters with lethal infections in largely the same way—with high morbidity (illness) and mortality (death) rates—and that as such, the history of disease among the native peoples of the New World, both before and after 1492, closely resembled the experiences of human populations in the rest of the world. Thus it challenges the widely held notion of New World exceptionalism, the belief that the experiences of native Americans with newly introduced diseases were more disastrous than those of Old World populations. This study also disputes popular images of a New World paradise, free of disease, hunger, and violence until germ-laden, rapacious Europeans began arriving on American shores after 1492. While these romantic notions have fueled the fantasies of many over the centuries, there is no evidence to support this interpretation; in fact, what evidence does exist clearly indicates that native Americans died as a result of disease, famine, and violence at rates similar to those experienced by their counterparts in the Old World. Furthermore, not only does rhetoric portraying an American Garden of Eden misrepresent reality, it does a great disservice to native Americans, both past and present. Romanticizing the lives of indigenous Americans reinforces a condescending paternalism and fosters a sort of reverse racism according to which, before 1492, the indigenous inhabitants of the New World lived in blissful harmony with one another and their environment, while people in other parts of the world, and Europeans in particular, killed each other at alarming rates and recklessly destroyed the natural environments in which they lived. The overall impact of this stereotyping has been to restrict the agency of native Americans because, in effect, it sets them and their world apart from and above the rest of humanity.[1]

During the past two decades, a growing number of scholars, myself included, have laid most of the blame for the catastrophic decline of native American populations on the introduction of previously unknown infections from the Old World. This book does not dispute the devastating impact of those diseases on the native societies of the New World, nor does it aim to minimize the extent of what one historian has termed "the greatest catastrophe in human history."[2] It does argue, however, that mortality owing to virgin soil epidemics of smallpox, measles, and plague was no higher in the Americas than it had been in Europe, Asia, and Africa when those same diseases first appeared there. This then raises several questions: If morbidity and mortality rates occasioned by the introduction of Old World diseases to the Americas were similar to those experienced by African, Asian, and European peoples, why was the outcome so different? After all, Africa, Asia, and Europe are still largely populated by people originally from those regions, while native Americans no longer make up the majority population in their homeland. Why did native American populations decline by 75 to 90 percent in the century following contact with Europeans? And perhaps more important: why did native American populations fail to recover as quickly and to the same extent as human populations in other parts of the world? Why did some indigenous people disappear altogether, while others struggled for centuries to recover only a fraction of their former numbers? And why were indigenous societies unable to regain political and economic autonomy over their homelands?

This study argues that it is the phenomenon of European colonialism as conceived and implemented by the four nations with the most extensive New World colonies, Spain, Portugal, France, and England, that explains the delayed or failed recovery of indigenous American populations. Throughout the colonial era, warfare and other forms of violence claimed the lives of significant numbers of natives; abusive labor practices, including slavery, significantly exacerbated indigenous mortality rates over the long term; and forced and voluntary migrations disrupted and ultimately undermined indigenous social, political, and economic institutions. It is not this author's intention, however, to present the reader with a detailed analysis of European imperialism and its myriad institutions; rather, this study focuses specifically on the points at which epidemic disease and colonialism intersected in the New World after 1492 and the consequences of those fateful junctures. To that end, this work concentrates on four central issues: first, the history of the human experience with epidemic disease in Europe, Africa, and Asia, and specifically how Old World peoples responded both biologically and culturally to outbreaks of epidemic illness before 1500; second, the nature of the disease environment of the Americas before 1492 as compared to that of the Old World; third, the history of the introduction of previously unknown disease organisms into the Americas after 1492 and the levels of morbidity and mortality occasioned by their arrival; and fourth, the relationship between the institutions and practices of European colonialism, epidemic disease, and demographic trends among native American populations throughout the hemisphere.

Since the early sixteenth century, many writers have expounded a variety of theories claiming to explain the stunning speed with which Europeans successfully colonized the Americas. For most of the last five hundred years, these arguments have tended to fall into three camps: those emphasizing the military skill, superior weaponry, and general perspicacity of Europeans; those attributing the victory of Europeans over native Americans to divine providence; and finally, those emphasizing the role European violence and brutality played in the subjugation and reduction of native populations. Until recently, the latter argument, dubbed The Black Legend, enjoyed especially wide acceptance.[3]

The origins of The Black Legend date to the earliest years of Spanish colonial rule. Throughout the sixteenth and seventeenth centuries, a number of writers, some of whom lived or traveled in the New World, recorded their impressions of the harshness of Spanish imperialism on the indigenous population. One of the most outspoken and possibly the best-known critic of Spanish colonialism was the Dominican friar Bartolomé de las Casas, who wrote several treatises on mistreatment of native Americans at the hands of Spanish officials and colonists. Las Casas's writings included many sensational descriptions of acts of Spanish cruelty perpetrated on the native populations of the Caribbean, Mexico, Central America, Venezuela, Colombia, Peru, and Florida. Typical of his descriptions is this account of Spanish atrocities on the island of Hispaniola:

> They forced their way into native settlements, slaughtering everyone they found there, including small children, old men, pregnant women, and even women who had just given birth. They hacked them to pieces, slicing open their bellies with their swords as though they were so many sheep herded into a pen. They even laid wagers on whether they could manage to slice a man in two at a stroke, or cut an individual's head from his body, or disembowel

him with a single blow of their axes. They grabbed suckling infants by the feet and, ripping them from their mothers' breasts, dashed them headlong against the rocks. Others, laughing and joking all the while, threw them over their shoulders into a river, shouting: "Wriggle, you little perisher."[4]

The inflammatory rhetoric of Las Casas proved politically expedient to the governments of rival European nations eager to tarnish Spain's image both at home and abroad, and as a result, the works of Las Casas and others similarly critical of Spanish imperialism were widely translated and circulated throughout Europe, reinforcing The Black Legend for centuries to come.

During the past three decades, however, another interpretation has held sway: that rather than European violence, virgin soil epidemics of virulent diseases introduced from the Old World explain the rapid die-off of native Americans and the subsequent success of European colonialism. Some, in fact, have gone as far as to argue that "since epidemics can account for virtually all of the extra mortality in the sixteenth century, the principle of Occam's razor suggests that it is not necessary to assume that there were other important causes of death. Thus, no reliance on the 'Black Legend' of Spanish homicide and cruelty is necessary to explain the observed population collapse."[5] It is this author's contention that because the role of epidemic disease was ignored for so long, during the past thirty years the pendulum has swung too far in that direction and scholars now overemphasize the long-term impact of disease and minimize the impact of other aspects of European colonialism. While it may not be the intention of these authors to do so, this emphasis on disease leaves readers with the distinct impression that other factors such as violence, slavery, and migration were not major contributing factors to the demographic decline of native American populations. This work is not a revival of The Black Legend, but rather an attempt to integrate the two views.

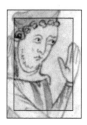

1 • Old World Epidemiology to 1500

The fact was that one citizen avoided another, that almost no one cared for his neighbor, and that relatives rarely or hardly ever visited each other—they stayed far apart. This disaster had struck such fear into the hearts of men and women that brother abandoned brother, uncle abandoned nephew, sister left brother, and very often wife abandoned husband, and—even worse, almost unbelievable—fathers and mothers neglected to tend and care for their children as if they were not their own.

What more can one say except that so great was the cruelty of Heaven, and, perhaps, also that of man, that from March to July of the same year [1348], between the fury of the pestiferous sickness and the fact that many of the sick were badly treated or abandoned in need because of the fear that the healthy had, more than one hundred thousand human beings are believed to have lost their lives for certain inside the walls of the city of Florence—whereas before the deadly plague, one would not even have estimated there were actually that many people dwelling in the city.

Giovanni Boccaccio, *The Decameron*

No people anywhere on earth at any time in human history have been able to avoid frequent and often fatal encounters with disease. In fact, illness and our responses to it constitute one of the great bonds joining us as human beings. And as the above passages illustrate, the terror and hopelessness experienced by individuals who have witnessed massive outbreaks of disease resonate centuries later and could just as easily have been written by someone observing the cholera pandemic of 1900, which claimed some 800,000 victims in India alone, or the present epidemic of AIDS, which has already infected more than 30 million people around the globe.

Outbreaks of disease that spread rapidly and affect large numbers of people within a community are termed epidemics; epidemics that range over a wide geographical area and affect an exceptionally high proportion of a population are sometimes labeled pandemics. Undoubtedly the best-known twentieth-century pandemic began in the spring of 1918, when an outbreak of influenza erupted in the United States. By the time the pandemic subsided a year later, more than 21 million people around the world had perished.

The term *virgin soil epidemic* describes the initial outbreak of a disease previously unknown or absent from a particular area for many generations; such events usually result in extremely high rates of morbidity and mortality. Virgin soil epidemics of measles, for example, routinely result in morbidity rates of over 90 percent, as was the case when measles first arrived among Pacific Islanders during the second half of the nineteenth century. When a virgin soil epidemic of measles struck the indigenous inhabitants of the Hawaiian Islands in 1848, it claimed the lives of 25 to 30 percent of the total population. Similarly, when measles first appeared in the Fiji Islands in 1875, 20 to 30 percent of the island's population perished within a period of several months.[1] Whenever virgin soil epidemics occur, the simultaneous illness and incapacitation of large numbers of individuals cause many serious problems: a decline or cessation in economic activities, including food production and distribution; the breakdown of political systems; and most important for sick individuals, the disruption of social service networks within families and communities. The sick require basic care—a regular supply of water, nourishment, and clean bedding. When such necessities are not available, the victim's condition can easily worsen, often resulting in death. When large numbers of the sick begin to die, economic, political, and social crises are magnified, as is the terror of the living who fear the loss of their own health, the loss of loved ones, and ultimately death itself.

That individuals and societies have always seen themselves as distinct from, and often superior to, others is a constant of human history. And this perception of difference, rather than similarity, and the conflicts it creates account for much of the turmoil and suffering in the human experience. But in the realm of biology, few such differences exist: all human populations show remarkable genetic similarity. In fact, geneticists claim that of the one hundred thousand human genes identified to

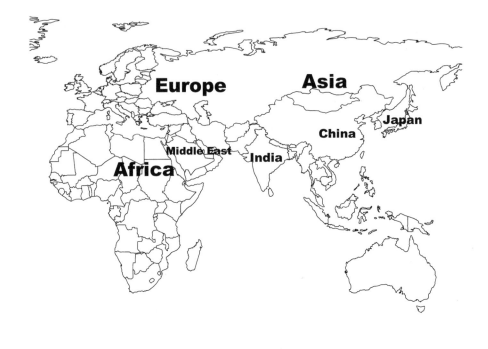

Map 1. *Regions of the Old World with Distinct Disease Patterns.*
Map by the author.

date, 99 percent are shared across human populations. So with regard to the biology of human life, many events, including birth, illness, and death, are truly universal.

Yet another area in which the universal character of the human condition manifests itself can be found in the biological and cultural responses of societies to epidemic disease. Although it is impossible to reconstruct completely the long and complicated history of relations between humans and disease, both archaeological and written sources provide us with enough information to arrive at three conclusions. First, while the responses of particular societies to epidemic disease differ in terms of such specifics as ceremonies of propitiation and remedies employed to cure the sick, in general the emotions experienced, the explanations offered, and the treatments/strategies adopted by affected populations around the world are strikingly similar. Second, massive epidemics of virulent infections posed an ongoing threat to the health and survival of human populations from at least 2000 BCE on. And in fact, disease became such an integral part of the human experience that, unless the outbreak was especially severe, historical records often failed to note its presence. Third, while mortality rates associated with virgin soil epidemics varied depending on the disease, its virulence, and the presence or absence of extenuating factors such as war or famine, the most devastating epidemics in human history have routinely claimed at least 20 to 40 percent of infected populations.

The Universal Nature of Human Responses to Disease

All traditional systems of medicine, whether they originated in East Asia, the Middle East, the Americas, Africa, or Europe, developed over many centuries with two express purposes. The first was preventative: to protect individuals and communities from illness. The second was curative: to aid those who had already succumbed to disease. How societies accomplished those goals varied from one region of the world to another, but in general, all subscribed to holistic theories that emphasized the need for balance and moderation in diet and behavior. And in fact, while some scholars argue that medical systems based on the classification and interpretation of bodily fluids and functions originated with the Greeks and Romans and were later adopted by Islamic societies, others argue convincingly that similar systems, albeit with slight variations, evolved independently in China, Japan, India, and the Americas. For example, according to Greek and Greco-Islamic texts, disease was caused by imbalances among the four humors—blood, phlegm, yellow bile, and black bile—which corresponded to four fundamental qualities—hot, cold, moist, and dry. Indian Ayurvedic medicine identified three humors, while the Chinese developed a similar system that identified heat, cold, humidity, dryness, and wind as causative agents of disease. In the Americas, native Andean medicine was based on an understanding of the three fluids of life—air, blood, and fat—as well as categories of hot and cold. Thus while each system has its own peculiarities, what is most striking are the similarities of classification and interpretation that developed independently in many areas of the world.[2]

Another feature common to all systems of traditional medicine is a reliance on drug therapy. Because of differences in local plant and animal materials available to medical practitioners, significant regional variations developed. Nevertheless, the philosophy behind the use of drug therapy remained the same—to prevent illness, to alleviate symptoms, and to cure the patient. In most parts of the world, local knowledge regarding herbal and other remedies was extensive; in China, for example,

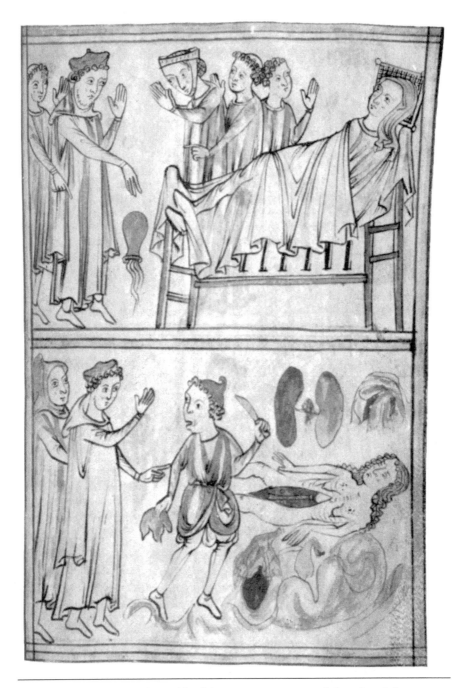

Fig. 1. *The universality of health-care practitioners: (above) a sick lady with her physician and (below) her postmortem, thirteenth century. (Bodleian Library, Oxford)*

physicians had described some 1,700 drugs by 1126 CE. An eleventh-century Islamic medical text identified more than 720 drugs, and Hindu medicine, which reached its zenith between the first and sixth centuries CE, employed a vast array of herbal cures.[3]

Another universal characteristic of human responses to ill health involved the explanation of disease causation. In all societies, divine or supernatural intervention was most often cited as the primary cause of disease. Islamic belief that the ultimate cause of illness was the will of God echoed the views of Christians, Confucians, Buddhists, Hindus, native Americans, and Africans. But while deities were ultimately responsible for visitations of disease, their arrival could also be linked to natural disasters, astrological events, and the breaking of social taboos. Traditional Chinese medicine ascribed the causation of disease to the wrath of dead ancestors who had to be placated by sacrifices or to demons who had to be exorcised from the body. Exorcism of disease by means of specialized ceremonies was also commonly practiced in many other societies and frequently supplemented drug therapies. Chinese Buddhists believed that "disease was the result of past sins, and recovery required the confession of these sins. . . . For each transgression, appropriate afflictions were imposed, and days were detracted from one's alloted lifetime."[4]

When bubonic plague struck the Middle East during the fourteenth century, many Moslems "believed that the plague was a punishment visited on man by God because they had strayed from the straight and narrow path of true belief."[5] And Boccaccio's dramatic description of the Florentine catastrophe in 1348 clearly placed responsibility for the epidemic on "the cruelty of Heaven, and, perhaps, also that of man."[6] Native Americans believed that "all illnesses were the result of biological and cosmic imbalances, [and] cures could be effected only by restoring the system to a state of equilibrium; and that required human intervention through the use of medicinal plants, rituals, and offerings to the gods."[7]

The strategies and responses of human populations to massive outbreaks of disease have also been remarkably similar. Because illness was so often attributed to divine providence, many societies developed ceremonies, sacrifices, and processions designed to appease the gods. In Christian communities one of the most common responses to the appearance of epidemic disease was the organization of religious processions during which clergy and laypeople removed the images of saints from their churches and carried them through the streets of the community, chanting and praying for divine mercy. During an epidemic in Paris in 1466, for example, thousands turned out to watch the remains of Saints Crepin and Crepinien being paraded through the streets.[8] Similarly, during an epidemic of smallpox that struck Japan in 993 CE, Buddhist monks

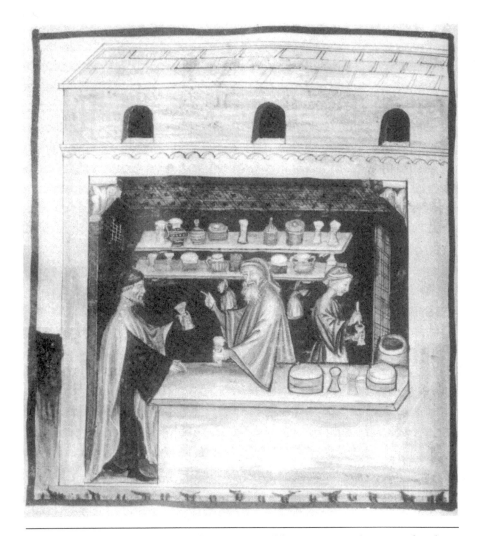

Fig. 2. *A fourteenth-century pharmacist and his customer. (Osterreichischen Nationalbibliothek, Vienna)*

and a crowd of several thousand organized a procession that marched to the coast in hopes of driving the disease out to sea.[9] Ironically, bringing large numbers of people together for public gatherings actually facilitated the spread of contagious illnesses and may, in fact, have worsened epidemics in many cases.

Among many subjects of the Inca empire of western South America, during epidemics, processions of armed men marched through their communities, attempting to drive out disease. But these processions also served a preventive function. Every year during the month of September people throughout the Inca empire celebrated *Citua,* one of the four most important festivals of the Inca calendar. Citua was an occasion for purification, "for it represented the expulsion from the city and the district of all the diseases and other ills and trouble that man can suffer."[10] In preparation for the festival, houses were washed and streets cleaned. After a period of fasting and sexual abstinence, families gathered to bathe and rub their bodies with bread, which absorbed illness and removed it from the body. At the same time in Cuzco, four members of the Inca royal family ran out from the center of the city, driving illness in front of them. The ceremony continued the next night, when torches were carried through the city for the same reason.[11]

Prayer was also an important and universal response to widespread outbreaks of illness, and many societies had prayers specifically written for such occasions. In India, prayers and offerings were directed to Shitala Mata, the Hindu goddess of smallpox. During outbreaks of plague in the Middle East in the fourteenth century, physicians directed their patients to repeat particular prayers a specific number of times each day: "Whoever repeated the various names of God, such as 'the Preserving' every day 896 times or 'the Vigilant' 312 times, would be safe. If a Muslim were devout and repeated 'the Subduer' over the ill 2142 times, plague would depart."[12]

In the face of epidemics, fear drove many to flee, sometimes, as noted by Boccaccio, abandoning home and family in the process. Islam expressly forbade flight from disease on the basis of three principles: "(1) plague was a mercy and a martyrdom from God for the faithful Muslim and a punishment for the infidel; (2) a Muslim should neither enter nor flee a plague-stricken land; and (3) there was no contagion of plague, because disease came directly from God."[13]

Nevertheless, during times of widespread sickness, many Moslems did flee. In 1348, for example, many Kurds in what is today southern Turkey fled the Black Death, as did the Mamluk Sultan, who fled Cairo on several occasions.[14] Certainly during the plague epidemics that ravaged Europe in the fourteenth century, flight was a common response, especially among members of the elite, who were widely criticized for their actions. In two English dioceses, for example, 20 percent of all priests abandoned their parishes during the Black Death.[15]

Another apparently widespread response to disease was the practice of isolation of the sick. Isolation could take several forms: the sick could be segregated alone or with their families, they could remain in their homes, or they could be removed to special facilities so that appropriate care could be given and they could not spread the illness to others. The first mention of isolation hospitals in Japan dates from the tenth century,

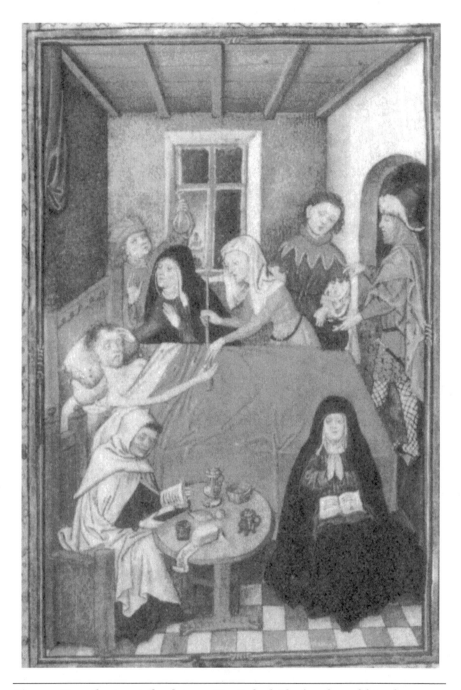

Fig. 3. *By gathering at the dying patient's bedside, family and friends facilitated the spread of contagious illness, about 1440. (Pierpont Morgan Library, New York)*

when epidemics of smallpox swept through the islands on six occasions.[16] In Europe isolation hospitals developed in response to the spread of leprosy between the eleventh and fourteenth centuries. In those communities where hospices were built, they were generally grim places where the sick went to die rather than recover. This is not surprising given the fact that before the twentieth century, rates of cure for serious illnesses were low. Even among Moslems who did not believe in the contagion of disease, hospitals were well established and funded by religious endowments at least by the thirteenth century. Over time, the function of European hospitals changed, and in addition to housing the sick and dying, they also became places for controlling and exploiting the poor.

In the end, what is most striking about the nature of human response to illness is its universal character. The frightening specter of disease elicited similar explanations of divine causality, similar systems of knowledge and classification, and similar responses, ranging from isolation of the sick and flight of the healthy to prayers and religious ceremonies designed either to drive out demons or to propitiate the gods. But despite the fact that human populations have developed remarkably similar sets of responses to illness, around the world communities faced distinctly different disease environments, each fraught with its own specific dangers.

The Origins and History of Human Disease in the Old World

Dating the origins of relations between humans and disease remains controversial and subject to constant backward revision. At the present time, most anthropologists agree that modern humans appeared in Africa sometime between 40,000 and 100,000 years ago. From there, they migrated into Asia and eventually Europe, the Americas, and Australia. Because early humans survived by hunting and gathering, constantly moving from one place to another, their numbers remained low. Small populations of hunter-gatherers could not support acute, epidemic diseases: both hosts and parasites would have been in danger of dying off. As a result, the diseases from which they suffered were probably endemic, meaning that after many generations of contact, these illnesses managed to establish themselves permanently among particular populations and as a result, they were present at low levels all year. They also tended to be relatively mild illnesses, often attacking young children with no previous exposure to the microorganism, rather than severe infections that affected everyone in a community. But even mild, low-grade infections could turn lethal if the host suffered stress as the result of injury or some other catastrophic event such as famine. In a weakened condition, the human body was unable to exist in equilibrium with its parasitic organisms, and death often ensued.

The extinction of large mammal species and the development of agriculture in various areas of the world between 12,000 and 15,000 years ago disrupted the equilibrium that had evolved between human hosts and disease organisms over thousands of years. Access to reliable supplies of food produced in central locations encouraged rapid growth of human populations, leading to increased alterations in the natural environment and changes in relations between humans and disease. Greater numbers of people, living first in rural communities and later in cities, produced large quantities of human wastes, contaminating water supplies and facilitating the spread of intestinal parasitic infections. The domestication of other animal species, and the close proximity in which they lived to humans, also affected disease patterns. Increased exposure to the infectious organisms of domesticated animals, including poultry, dogs, cattle, mice, rats, pigs, horses, sheep, cats, and goats, resulted in the transfer of these organisms to humans. In fact, more than 250 of the diseases with which humans have had long-standing relations originated in other species. For example, smallpox is closely related to and probably descended from cowpox or possibly monkey pox; measles is probably related to rinderpest, a disease that infects cattle as well as sheep and goats; the bacilli causing human, bovine, and avian tuberculosis are remarkably similar; and influenza viruses are found among populations of hogs, fowl, horses, and humans.[17]

At least by 4000 BCE, the growth of human populations led to the development of complex societies in various regions of North Africa, Asia, and India. Along with civilization and the concentration of large numbers of people within circumscribed areas came contact with new types of diseases, especially bacterial and viral infections that passed directly from one human to another. Because individuals who contracted crowd-type diseases either died as a result or acquired varying degrees of immunity, these organisms required large numbers of non-immune individuals in order to sustain themselves within a particular population. Thus in densely settled areas, migrants from the countryside or people from newly conquered territories provided a constant supply of fuel for disease organisms such as the smallpox virus and the bacteria responsible for causing pneumonia.

During the next 3000 to 4000 years, patterns of disease specific to particular civilizations developed. While painful and often costly in terms of human lives in the short run, civilized populations acquired extensive experience with a myriad of infections, conferring a significant advantage over their less immunologically advanced neighbors. When expanding into new territories, hordes of migrants and imperial armies traveled with powerful, invisible allies—infectious diseases with which neighboring populations often had little or no experience. Thus migration and colonization became the driving forces behind the spread of disease from one area of the globe to another, a process that only accelerated during the twentieth century due to advances in transportation technology, especially air travel.

By the beginning of the Christian era, each of the four major areas of civilization in the Old World, the Middle East, India, China, and the Mediterranean, had evolved their own unique patterns of disease. Unfortunately, a lack of evidence and/or scholarly research hampers our knowledge of the early history of particular diseases in many regions of the world, especially those outside of Europe. Compared to the paucity of scholarship on the history of disease in Africa in particular and to a lesser extent on Asia and the Middle East, the amount of information on European epidemics is relatively abundant and as a result, the history of disease in Europe is better understood and more accessible.

Nevertheless, archaeological and documentary evidence indicates that the disease patterns of the Middle East and India were probably the oldest and, therefore, the most stable of the four. In the Middle East, archaeological evidence indicates that before the Christian era, humans suffered from a variety of ills, including dysentery, typhoid and paratyphoid fevers, tuberculosis, polio, and various parasitic infections, some of them serious. In addition, leprosy had become increasingly common by the early centuries of the Christian era.[18] The oldest references to epidemic disease yet discovered come from the Middle East, where ancient texts recorded epidemics at least by 2000 BCE, and archaeologists have discovered three Egyptian mummies from the Eighteenth and Twentieth Dynasties (1570–1085 BCE) showing clear signs of smallpox pustules. In addition, cuneiform tablets from the Hittite Empire, located in present-day Turkey, described a serious outbreak of contagious disease, possibly smallpox, that decimated the Hittites sometime in the middle of the fourteenth century BCE. An accurate description of the disease was recorded in 302 CE, and regular references to epidemics of smallpox began to appear after 600 CE.

In tenth-century Baghdad, the Persian-born physician Rhazes recorded a detailed description of the illness:

> The outbreak of smallpox is preceded by continuous fever, aching in the back, itching in the nose and shivering during sleep. The main symptoms of its presence are: backache with fever, stinging pain in the whole body, congestion of the face, sometimes shrinkage, violent redness of the cheeks and eyes, a sense of pressure in the body, creeping of the flesh, pain in the throat and breast accompanied by difficulties of respiration and coughing, dryness of the mouth, thick salivation, hoarseness of the voice,

headache and pressure in the head, excitement, anxiety, nausea and unrest.[19]

Rhazes as well as other Islamic physicians clearly distinguished between smallpox and measles, indicating that the latter disease was also long established in the region. Inoculation, the process of introducing a small amount of the smallpox virus into the body of a healthy individual in order to stimulate the production of antibodies, was practiced in Egypt at least by the thirteenth century and probably had been introduced from India.

The history of smallpox in Africa remains vague, but it seems likely that trans-Saharan caravans introduced the disease into densely populated West Africa by the eighth century. No documentary evidence records its arrival, but the disease undoubtedly took a heavy toll on several genera-

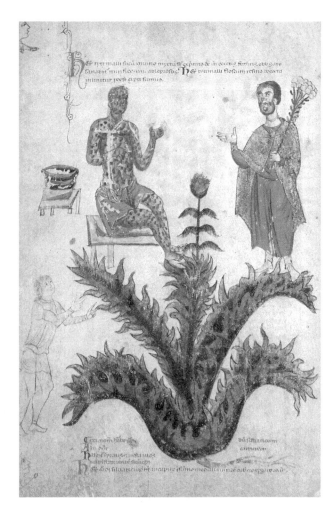

Fig. 4.
A physician confers with a patient suffering from a severe infection of the skin, possibly leprosy or smallpox. (Codex Vindobonensis 93, Osterreichischen Nationalbibliothek, Vienna)

tions of West Africans following its first outbreak. In East Africa, traders from India and Arabia probably introduced smallpox by the thirteenth or fourteenth centuries. Evidence reveals that as late as the seventeenth century, all segments of the population, adults as well as children, were still succumbing to the illness, indicating that smallpox was not yet endemic in the area:

> The fourth affliction and trouble that overtook this Kaffraria [the region of the Kaffirs, a population of South African Bantu speakers] was a severe outbreak of smallpox, of which a great number of people died. This disease along the whole of the coast is like a subtle pestilence, as it kills everyone in a house where it appears, men, women, and children alike, and very few escape who are attacked by it, as they do not know of a cure. . . . This smallpox is not infectious to Portuguese, except to children of tender-age, even though they hold intercourse with Kaffirs suffering from it.[20]

Of all the regions of the world, the history of disease in sub-Saharan Africa, before European colonization at the end of the nineteenth century, is probably the least understood, owing to a paucity of documentary and archaeological evidence and, until recently, a lack of interested researchers. But as research findings emerge, it is clear that for thousands of years, Africans coexisted with a variety of disease-causing organisms, including arboviruses such as dengue and yellow fever; trypanomiasis, or African sleeping sickness; yaws; leprosy; typhoid fever; dysentery; and a variety of parasitic infections, many of them serious. In addition to introducing smallpox, contact with Indian and Middle Eastern traders probably also resulted in the arrival of measles and chicken pox into sub-Saharan Africa several centuries ago. It is interesting to note that syphilis, bacterial pneumonia, and tuberculosis were rare or nonexistent before European colonization, but coincident with intensive European settlement, all three became serious threats to public health in the 1860s.[21]

While historians have yet to uncover archaeological evidence relating to India's earliest outbreaks of disease, this region possessed both the tropical climate and dense human population necessary for the propagation of acute, epidemic illness. It is known that typhoid fever, malaria, leprosy, pneumonia, dysentery, tuberculosis, and parasitic infections were common in the pre-Christian era. The origins of bubonic plague are not clear, but it appears likely that plague also had ancient roots on the Indian subcontinent. Cholera, another disease widely associated with India, was well established there at least by the beginning of the Christian era.[22]

As was true in Egypt, smallpox appears to have been present in India by at least 1500 BCE. A traditional medical text written sometime before 400 CE described the disease and explained its humoral etiology:

> Before *Masurika* [smallpox] fever occurs, with pain over the body, but particularly in the back. . . . The pustules are red, yellow, and white and they are accompanied with burning pain. The pustules become black and flat, are depressed in the centre, with much pain. They ripen slowly. . . . This form is cured with much difficulty, and it is called *Charmo* or fatal form.[23]

The long history of this disease in India is also supported by widespread worship of the goddess of smallpox, Shitala Mata, "the cool one," a possible reference to the popular treatment of cooling patients suffering from the high fever associated with the illness. In addition, documentary evidence suggests Indians practiced inoculation against the disease as early as the first millennium BCE.[24] While scattered references to the disease exist, detailed descriptions of epidemics do not appear until the sixteenth century.

Epidemics of smallpox, measles, and other infectious diseases regularly struck communities in India and the Middle East from at least 2000 BCE on, but their arrival in China and Europe was delayed by geographic isolation and low population density respectively. As a result, Chinese and European populations had less experience with specific infectious diseases. In China, influenza, malarial fevers, pneumonia, tuberculosis, and other pulmonary infections were present by the first millennium BCE.[25] The Huns, invading from central Asia, probably introduced smallpox into northern China around 250 BCE, and it had become endemic in that region by the beginning of the Christian era. Smallpox arrived in southern China by at least 48 CE, possibly as a result of increased trade with merchants from India, Central Asia, and the Middle East. By the sixth century CE, the disease was well established in China, and worship of a goddess of smallpox was widespread at least by the eleventh century.[26] Also by that time, Chinese physicians possessed sufficient experience with infectious diseases to be able to distinguish between smallpox, chicken pox, measles, and scarlet fever. Inoculation, practiced by the eleventh century and possibly as early as the second century, was probably introduced from India. Certainly preventive use of inoculation was widespread in China by the sixteenth century.[27]

In spite of its geographic isolation from the disease pools of India and the Middle East, at least 130 epidemics were recorded in various parts of China between the first century CE and 1500. Evidence does not allow for

Table 1.1 Mortality Associated with Epidemics in the Old World before 1500

Location	Date	Disease	Mortality	Source
Athens	430 BCE	smallpox	one-quarter of the Athenian army and countless civilians died	Thucydides, 118
Roman Empire	165–180 CE	smallpox	25–33 percent of infected population died; 3.5–7 million died	McNeill, 116; Hopkins, 22–23
Egypt	165–180 CE	smallpox	30–90 percent decline in number of male taxpayers in several communities	Duncan-Jones, 20–21
Constanti-nople	541–542 CE	bubonic plague	40 percent of total population; 10,000 deaths per day in the city	Hopkins, 23
Mediter-ranean region	6th and 7th centuries	bubonic plague	population reduced by 40–60 percent	Gottfried (1983), 11–12
Izumi Province, Japan	735–737 CE	smallpox	44 percent of adult population died; 25–35 percent of the total population died	Farris, 378–81
Japan	812–814 CE	smallpox	"almost half" of the population died	Farris, 378–81
Cairo	1347–1349	Black Death/ bubonic plague	between one-third and one-half of the population (200,000 people) died	Watts, 25–26
"some cities and villages" in England and Italy	1348–1400	Black Death/ bubonic plague	70–80 percent died	Herlihy (1997), 17
Europe	1348–1420	Black Death/ bubonic plague	total population reduced by 30–60 percent	Herlihy (1997), 17; Slack, 15

reliable diagnoses of the infections involved, although smallpox and measles were probably involved in many instances, but a number of documents include descriptions of the regions affected as well as estimates of mortality. As table 2 reveals, in at least fifteen instances, the number of deaths reached 20 percent and often much higher. Indeed, mortality rates of 30 to 60 percent and more occurred on a number of occasions.

Because of close geographical, religious, and cultural ties, the history of infectious diseases in Japan closely parallels that of China, although the chronology of epidemics in Japan tends to be later because many illnesses arrived first in China and later spread to the islands of Japan. For example, evidence indicates that smallpox was introduced to Japan from China during the sixth century, coincident with the spread of Buddhism to the islands from the mainland. The first recorded epidemic of that disease raged between 735 and 737, claiming 44 percent of the adult population of the province of Izumi. Overall, 25 to 35 percent of the Japanese population died during this three-year period. Another massive outbreak in 812–814 reportedly claimed "almost half" of the population. In both instances, rapid demographic decline led to severe political, economic, and social crises.[28] Official court records indicate that from the eighth to the tenth centuries, epidemics occurred on average every three to four years. It is no wonder, then, that one scholar has dubbed the period from 700 to 1050 "The Age of Plagues." By the thirteenth century, outbreaks of smallpox had become fewer and less frequent, suggesting that the disease had become endemic.[29]

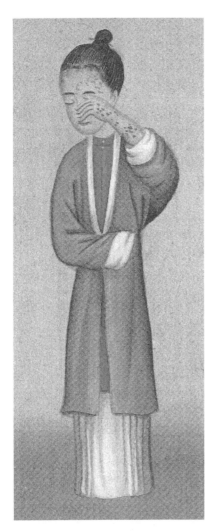

Accounts of smallpox from the Southeast Asian islands of Borneo and the Philippines do not appear until the sixteenth century, but it seems likely that the disease arrived there some centuries before. Thus by the beginning of the Christian era, smallpox had a long history in India and the Middle East and was on its way to becoming endemic in

Fig. 5. *China: A young girl, possibly suffering from smallpox or measles. (Bibliothèque Nationale, Paris)*

Table 1.2 Epidemics in China, 16–1500 CE

Location	Date (CE)	Mortality
Southern China—military engagement	16	60–70 percent of troops died
Mongolia—famine and epidemic	46	two-thirds died
Sinkiang and Kokonor—military engagement	162	30–40 percent of troops died
Hupeh—military engagement—famine and epidemic	208	two-thirds of troops died
northern and central China—locusts and famine precede epidemic	312	"in Shensi only one or two out of a hundred taxpayers survived"
undefined	322	20–30 percent died
Shantung	762	more than one-half died
Chekiang	806	more than one-half died
Hupeh, Kiangsu, Anhui	891	30–40 percent died
Honan	1232	"90,000 died in less than 50 days"
Hopei	1331	90 percent died
Shansi, Hopei, Kiangsi—military engagement	1351–1352	50 percent of troops died
Hupeh, Kiangsi, Shansi, Suiyuan	1353	in Shansi more than two-thirds died
Shansi, Hupeh, Hopei, Kiangsi, Hunan, Kwangtung, Kwangsi	1354	in Hupeh 60–70 percent died
Hunan	1489	"whole villages and towns perished"

Source: McNeill, Plagues and Peoples (1976), 260–69.

China, all regions with dense populations. But populations in Europe and Africa south of the Sahara were too small and widely separated at that time to have supported the illness. So the disease died out after major outbreaks, sometimes for centuries, only to flare again when smallpox was reintroduced from the outside.

Compared to the antiquity of epidemics in India and the Middle East, the history of massive outbreaks of infectious diseases in Europe appears to be more recent. Archaeological evidence indicates that at least by the first millennium BCE, pneumonia, tuberculosis, poliomyelitis, dysentery, diphtheria, and malaria, as well as other illnesses, were well established among European populations.[30] But the earliest description of a massive epidemic dates from Athens in the fourth century BCE. According to the

Greek historian Thucydides, the epidemic began in 430 BCE during the Peloponnesian War:

> Not many days after their arrival in Attica the plague first began to show itself among the Athenians. It was said that it had broken out in many places previously in the neighborhood of Lemnos and elsewhere; but a pestilence of such extent and mortality was nowhere remembered. Neither were the physicians at first of any service, ignorant as they were of the proper way to treat it, but they died themselves the most thickly, as they visited the sick most often; nor did any human art succeed any better. Supplications in the temples, divinations, and so forth were found equally futile, till the overwhelming nature of the disaster at last put a stop to them altogether.[31]

Thucydides reported that the disease originated in Ethiopia, spreading from there into Egypt and Libya, and his vivid description of the fever and pustules characteristic of this outbreak leaves little doubt that the disease responsible for the devastation was smallpox. The epidemic lasted two to three years, during which time it claimed the lives of one-quarter of the Athenian army and countless civilians.[32] Another epidemic of smallpox broke out in the Greek city of Syracuse in 395 BCE;

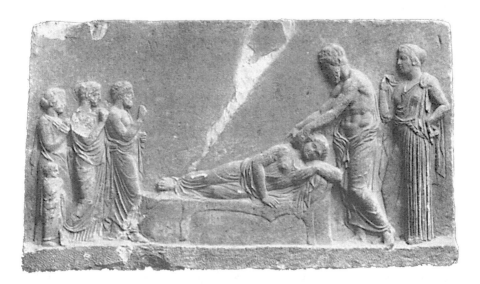

Fig 6. *The Greek god of healing, Asklepios, cures a sleeping woman, early fourth century BCE. (Deutsches Archaeologisches Institut, Athens)*

this incident too was reported to have originated in Libya.[33] From Greece, smallpox could have spread north and west into central Europe, but no evidence of such a development exists.

The next recorded incidence of smallpox in Europe occurred in Italy in 164 or 165 CE. The Plague of Antonius, as it was called, first appeared among Roman soldiers returning from Syria. The disease spread quickly throughout Italy and reportedly claimed as many as 2,000 lives per day in Rome. From there, the epidemic moved into other parts of the Roman Empire, where it raged for some fifteen years. Estimates of the mortality during this prolonged outbreak range from 3.5 million to 7 million throughout the empire.[34]

By the sixth century, smallpox was becoming increasingly common in various regions of Europe. In 580–581, the disease spread across southern France and northern Italy, claiming many lives.[35]

But while isolated outbreaks were also recorded in France and on the Iberian Peninsula during the late seventh and eleventh centuries, the disease appears to have retreated from many areas of the continent. The Crusades of the twelfth and thirteenth centuries facilitated the reintroduction of smallpox from the Middle East throughout Europe, and by the end of the twelfth century, the disease was becoming increasingly common, and less virulent, throughout the continent.[36]

Twentieth-century research on the smallpox virus confirms that the organism is, like many viruses, extremely mutable. Thus the virulence of smallpox has waxed and waned during the many centuries that it has made its home among human populations. Certainly in much of the Old World at least by the fourteenth century, smallpox was an endemic and relatively mild childhood infection, one that conferred lifelong immunity on its victims. But according to medical historians Ann Carmichael and Arthur Silverstein, by the second half of the sixteenth century, the disease had taken on a renewed virulence. The first recorded outbreak of the newly lethal strain of the infection appeared in Naples in 1544. Thirty years later, "eight major epidemics of smallpox were reported, with additional descriptions of malignant pustules and high childhood mortality that began to resemble the *Variola major* of the next two centuries."[37]

From the sixth century until the reappearance of virulent smallpox in the sixteenth century, influenza, leprosy, tuberculosis, and bubonic plague constituted the infections most feared by European populations. Influenza is a highly contagious respiratory illness. While the infection probably appeared much earlier in human history, the first recorded European epidemic may have occurred in Italy, Germany, and England in 1173, followed by additional outbreaks in Italy and France in 1323. The number of epidemics increased during the fifteenth century, with incidents in Paris in

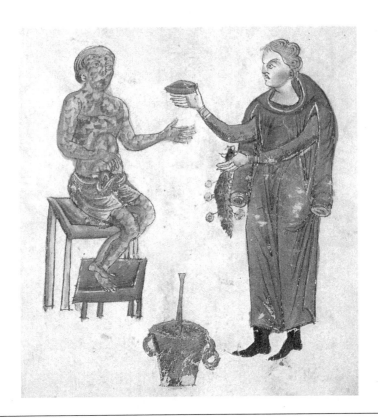

Fig. 7. *A physician administering medicine to a patient covered with sores. (Codex Vindobonensis 93, Osterreichischen Nationalbibliothek, Vienna)*

1411, 1414, and 1427. The infamous English "sweating sickness," which first appeared in 1485 and returned in 1508, 1517, 1528, and 1551, was also probably caused by the influenza virus.[38] One of the most dreaded diseases of the Middle Ages was leprosy, which appeared in historical records throughout western Europe with increasing frequency during the eleventh to fourteenth centuries. While skeletal evidence indicates that cases of leprosy did in fact occur in Europe, many of those diagnosed with the disease were probably suffering from other ills. Origins of the disease are obscure, but it may have been introduced from India and spread throughout the continent by Roman colonization. Certainly it was well known in France as early as 635, when the Lombard king Rothari codified policy for dealing with victims of the illness:

> If anyone is affected with leprosy and the truth of the matter is
> recognized by the judge or by the people and the leper is expelled

from the civitas or from the house so that he lives alone, he shall not have the right to alienate his property or to give it to anyone because on the day he is expelled from the home it is as if he had died. Nevertheless, while he lives, he should be nourished on the income from that which remains.[39]

The spread of this disfiguring disease prompted the construction of thousands of "leprosy houses" or hospitals throughout Europe between 1090 and 1260.[40]

By the eleventh century, western European elites were using the diagnosis of leprosy, accompanied by its stigma and attendant loss of personal property and freedom, as a form of social and political control in order to persecute individuals perceived as deviants, especially Jews, heretics, and witches. In addition to being expelled from civil society, lepers were often forced to wear special clothing and carry a bell or clapper to warn strangers to keep their distance. In France and Spain, the persecution of lepers culminated in a series of massacres in 1321.[41] The number of reported cases of leprosy declined steadily during the fourteenth and fifteenth centuries in part because massacres and epidemics of bubonic plague had significantly reduced the population of lepers. Even more important, however, was the increased incidence of a closely related disease, tuberculosis. Both leprosy and tuberculosis are caused by bacilli, and exposure to tuberculosis appears to confer limited immunity to leprosy. Because tuberculosis is transferred more easily, via droplets dispersed by coughing and sneezing, this disease spread more quickly and was gradually able to displace leprosy.[42]

The increased incidence of epidemics in Europe and China during the first thousand years of the present era was directly related to expanding trade networks between Old World civilizations. Disease organisms traveled both by land and by sea along the major trade routes between Asia, Europe, and the Middle East. As a result, by at least 1000 CE, humans in the Old World lived in a unified and relatively stable disease environment. Epidemics occurred periodically, but the diseases themselves became less virulent as time passed and immunities increased. Over the course of many generations, most of these became diseases of childhood, illnesses that young people contracted and from which they recovered, usually with little or no serious complications. This is not to say that large numbers of people, especially infants and children, were not dying annually of infectious diseases—they were. But relative to the virulence of epidemics and high rates of mortality that preceded and followed this period, humans enjoyed a respite from the most serious depredations of disease.

All of this changed, however, around 1200 CE, with the expansion of the Asian caravan trade, the rise of the Mongol Empire, and the creation of new commercial routes across the Eurasian steppe between China and Russia. As merchants and Mongol armies traversed northern Eurasia, their traveling companions, Indian black rats and their fleas, introduced the bacilli that cause bubonic plague to the rodent population of that region. The ferocity of the epidemics that followed so devastated the populations of Europe and the Middle East that the "Black Death," as it came to be known, has occupied a central place in the collective memory of those populations for the past six centuries.[43]

The first recorded epidemic of bubonic plague probably originated in eastern Africa, spreading throughout the Mediterranean Basin in 541–542. Named after the Byzantine emperor of the time, the Plague of Justinian claimed up to ten thousand lives daily in Constantinople and eventually reduced the population of that city by approximately 40 percent before moving west into Italy, France, Germany, Spain, and England. At least one description also included references to "blisters the size of a lentil," suggesting the presence of smallpox.[44] According to the Byzantine court historian, Procopius:

> During this time there was a pestilence, by which the whole human race came near to being annihilated. . . . It started from the Egyptians who dwell in Pelusium. Then it divided and moved in one direction towards Alexandria and the rest of Egypt and in other directions; it came to Palestine on the borders of Egypt and from here it spread over the whole world, always moving forward and traveling at times favorable to it.[45]

The disease reappeared frequently in the Mediterranean area throughout the sixth and seventh centuries, reducing the population of that region by 40 to 60 percent. By the end of the eighth century, however, plague appears to have disappeared entirely from the region.[46] The history of bubonic plague in China remains unclear, but limited evidence suggests that the disease may have struck Chinese populations during the seventh and eighth centuries, possibly returning again during the twelfth through fourteenth centuries.[47] In India, the first documented outbreak occurred in 1812, but it seems likely that serious epidemics in 1443, 1548, 1573, 1590, and 1618 may have been caused by the disease.[48]

The prolonged absence of bubonic plague from Europe and the Middle East for many generations explains, at least in part, the exceptionally high mortality rates of the fourteenth century. The other factor contributing to the catastrophic number of deaths was that in addition to bubonic plague, characterized by the appearance of buboes, or areas of swelling, contemporary sources indicate that the even more lethal septicemic, or blood-borne, and pneumonic, or airborne, forms of the disease were also present. Even today, mortality from the latter two infections is almost always 100 percent.

While several scholars have claimed that the plague pandemics of the fourteenth century originated in China, the evidence is far from clear.[49] In any event, the arrival of the Black Death in the region of the Crimea in 1346–1347 is indisputable. From this central location, the disease traveled in two directions: south and east into the Middle East and west and north into Europe. By 1348, plague had traveled as far west as the Iberian Peninsula, and one year later it struck the populations of the British Isles, France, and Scandinavia. By the time the pandemic subsided seven years later, in 1353, it had doubled back to the east, arriving in Moscow in the summer of that year.[50] All told, this initial outbreak of plague probably claimed between one-third and two-thirds of Europe's population, and according to one estimate, between 1348 and 1400, many communities in England and Italy lost 70 to 80 percent of their populations to the Black Death.[51] Epidemics of plague flared again in the 1360s and 1370s, although with decreased virulence. Thereafter the disease continued to appear throughout Europe at least every twenty-five years until the end of the seventeenth century, when it finally receded once again.

During the fourteenth and fifteenth centuries, outbreaks of plague posed a serious threat to the survival of local societies and economies. Soaring mortality rates reduced the number of workers in all sectors of the economy, and as a result, the production of food and other commodities declined dramatically. Not surprisingly, famine often followed in the wake of plague, claiming the lives of many more. In Cairo, for example, between one-third and one-half of the population, some two hundred thousand people, died of plague between 1347 and 1349. In rural areas surrounding the city, the deaths of thousands of peasants and the flight of many more led to grain shortages and famine. Starvation further reduced the population, and so both the agricultural and textile-manufacturing sectors collapsed. Fifty years later, Egyptian agricultural production remained significantly lower than it had been before the Black Death, illustrating the long-term impact of this demographic disaster.[52]

But while the immediate consequences of the Black Death affected European and Middle Eastern populations equally, the responses of local elites to crises of public health differed significantly and ultimately influenced the frequency and severity of future epidemics. Especially after 1450, European elites devised a series of controls that significantly reduced mortality and eventually the number of outbreaks as well. The key to preventing the spread of plague was controlling the movements of people. Thus policies first implemented in northern Italy enforced quarantines on areas suspected of harboring the disease, isolated the sick and their families either in their homes or in plague hospitals, compelled burials of those who had died of the disease as well as the destruction of their personal property, and provided assistance both to those isolated within their homes and those whose livelihoods were disrupted by market closures. Peasants and the urban poor often objected to quarantines and the destruction of their meager belongings, but in the end, local authorities prevailed. The result of the successful imposition of plague controls throughout much of western Europe was twofold: it strengthened the power of local and national elites, and it hastened the decline and eventual disappearance of plague from the region between 1450 and 1650.[53]

In the Middle East, on the other hand, plague continued to pose a serious threat to public health until the early nineteenth century. Because Moslems regarded the disease as the will of God, and because those who died of plague went to paradise, both Mamluk and Ottoman officials failed to devise specific policies aimed at preventing the spread of epidemics. Finally after 1844, plague receded from Egypt and much of the region as a result of the adoption of European public health measures by the Mamluk ruler of Egypt, Muhammad Ali.[54]

While the immediate demographic consequences of the Black Death devastated European societies, in the long run, they may have produced important benefits. Historian David Herlihy has argued that epidemics of plague in the fourteenth and fifteenth centuries undermined the social and economic systems, characterized by "high population density, intensive grain production, and widespread poverty," that had developed during the Middle Ages.[55] The severe labor shortages that followed eventually led to higher wages for the poor and the development of new technologies. In addition, the poor gradually adopted elite strategies for limiting family size, especially postponing marriage, thus ensuring that rapid population recovery did not undermine their recent economic advance.

The Significance of the Old World Disease Experience

In spite of the large gaps that exist in our understanding of the evolution of the relationship between humans and disease, especially for regions outside of Europe, several conclusions emerge. First, epidemics occurred frequently throughout the Old World before 1500. In the Roman Empire, between 490 and 165 BCE, for example, outbreaks of infectious diseases occurred every four to eight years.[56] In Japan, between the eighth and tenth centuries, epidemics occurred every three to four years on average.[57] And

beginning as early as 7000 BCE. "Diffusionists," as those who argue that intentional contacts between the Old and New Worlds took place long before the end of the fifteenth century are known, argue that before 1492, the Americas were not the biologically and culturally isolated regions long described by many archaeologists and other academics, but rather a crossroads for exploratory expeditions from civilizations as diverse as Shang Dynasty China (1100 BCE) and Bronze Age Scandinavia (800 BCE). Recently a growing number of researchers have begun to concede some legitimacy to the claims of the diffusionists, but they continue to minimize the impact of what one scholar has termed "ephemeral contacts."[2]

Many generations passed as waves of migratory groups slowly made their way south, but archaeological evidence indicates that by 9000 BCE, human populations had reached the tip of South America. Throughout the American continent, indigenous populations developed in significantly different ways in response to the environments in which they settled. It is

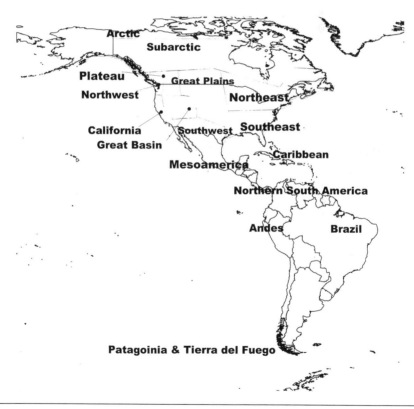

Map 2. *Regions of the Americas. Map by the author.*

important to remember that the native peoples Europeans encountered were often only the latest in a long series of societies inhabiting specific regions. As such, these societies had inherited the cultural and technological achievements of generations of people who had preceded them. In central Mexico, for example, the Mexica, often referred to as the Aztecs, built their empire upon the cultural foundations of their predecessors, who included the Olmecs, Zapotecs, Mixtecs, Toltecs, Totonacs, and many others. Similarly, the roots of Maya civilization in southern Mexico and northern Central America stretch far back into the Archaic past. And in the Andes, the Inca empire emerged from an amalgam of social, political, and economic features derived from its predecessors, including the Nazca, Mochica, Chimu, and Huari.

Health and Disease Before 1492

The Incas, rulers, commoners, as well as the ancient people of these kingdoms, lived long and healthy lives, many reaching the age of 150 to 200 years because they had an ordered and methodical regimen for living and eating.[3]

There was then no sickness; they had no aching bones; they had then no high fever; they had then no smallpox; they had then no burning chest; they had then no abdominal pain; they had then no consumption; they had then no headache. At that time the course of humanity was orderly. The foreigners made it otherwise when they arrived here.[4]

The preceding passages, the first by a seventeenth-century Inca chronicler, the second by an oft-quoted eighteenth-century Maya, paint an idyllic picture of native life and health in the Americas before the arrival of Europeans. According to these authors, before the beginning of the sixteenth century, no serious diseases ravaged native populations, people consumed a balanced diet, and as a result, many individuals lived long, healthy lives. Other New World peoples also remember precolonial times as halcyon days when life was longer and happier.[5] But according to many native writers, beginning in 1492 this earthly paradise was shattered forever by the arrival of conquistadors, colonists, and microbes from the Old World. From one end of the Americas to the other, native societies reeled under the exactions of European colonialism and the onslaught of virgin soil epidemics of smallpox, measles, and bubonic plague.

Because the suffering and mortality occasioned by these epidemics was so great, one can easily understand why native writers looked back on the past as a time relatively free of disease, and ultimately as a time when people's lives were longer and happier. While this tendency to romanticize life in the Americas before 1492 may be understandable, reality was much more complex. During the last twenty years, a growing number of scholars have begun to challenge the image of the precontact paradise enshrined in native lore. Nevertheless, some have continued to perpetuate this myth, painting a uniquely benign portrait of the disease environment of the New World.[6] But with advances in paleopathology and paleodemography, a very different picture of the length and quality of life in pre-Columbian America has emerged. And given the genetic similarity of all human populations, it should come as no surprise that in spite of their relative isolation from the rest of the world, epidemics, famines, and wars occurred with regularity throughout the hemisphere before the arrival of Europeans, reducing life expectancies and raising mortality rates. In fact, far from an earthly paradise, the profile that emerges of life and death in the New World resembles that of the Old in several important respects.

Our knowledge of human mortality in the pre-Columbian Americas comes from a variety of sources. Native chroniclers such as Felipe Guaman Poma de Ayala and Garcilaso de la Vega and the Mexica physician Martin de la Cruz recorded a wealth of information concerning all aspects of life in Inca and Mexica society. Their descriptions of health and disease before the arrival of Europeans reveal the occurrence of devastating epidemics, famines, and wars. Guaman Poma, for example, attributed the Inca conquest of the Indian societies of northern Chile to "the ravages of plague, which lasted for ten years." He also alluded to other periods of epidemic disease, famine, war, and natural disasters.[7] In addition, the writings of colonial European observers such as Father Pablo Joseph de Arriaga in Peru and Father Bernardino de Sahagún in Mexico provide much useful data on disease, healing, and death. According to Sahagún's chronology of the Mexica rulers of Tenochtitlán:

> Moctezuma the Elder was fifth [1440–1469], and ruled Tenochtitlán thirty years. He conquered and made war on all the people of Chalco; and on Quauhnauc and on all who were subject to Quauhnauc; and Macauacan. And in his reign there came a great famine, which spread over the land for four years.[8]

While colonial documents are useful for establishing the existence of epidemics, famines, and wars, and while they sometimes contain information on timing and even vague descriptions of the degree of mortality, with regard to disease they do not provide sufficient information to determine with certainty the cause of these incidents.

But recent discoveries in the fields of paleopathology and paleodemography are revealing valuable data about life and death in the pre-Columbian Americas. During the last twenty years, the number of prehistoric sites surveyed for skeletal materials has expanded rapidly. This, combined with the development of new techniques of chemical and biomechanical analysis, including stable isotope ratios of carbon and nitrogen and DNA analysis, allows paleopathologists and bioarchaeologists to arrive at a clearer understanding of dietary and disease patterns.[9] In many instances, skeletal materials reveal unmistakable signs of illness, nutritional deficiencies, and violence. Disruptions in bone growth, called Harris lines, suggest periods of acute physiological stress caused by disease or malnutrition. Likewise, disruptions in the formation of tooth enamel, Wilson's bands, indicate periods of physical distress, while a high incidence of dental caries suggests a diet overly dependent on carbohydrates, probably corn.

Skeletal remains from prehistoric burial sites also reveal valuable information on the level of mortality in particular societies. For example, mortuary evidence from Teotihuacan, the wealthy and powerful Classic-period (150 BC–750 CE) city situated north of Mexico City, indicates mortality rates as high or higher than those of European cities in the preindustrial era. Infants and children succumbed in especially large numbers, and as a result, the city's population maintained or expanded only as a result of in-migration.[10]

But despite advances in research, serious problems remain with skeletal analysis. First, many infections leave no trace on human bones; in fact, most acute, epidemic diseases leave no specific marker because the human host either dies or recovers before any serious skeletal damage can take place. Furthermore, most infectious diseases affect soft tissue, and except for a few notable exceptions in extremely dry areas of the southwestern United States and coastal Peru and Ecuador, soft tissue remains are scarce. Those diseases affecting the human skeleton are often chronic bacterial infections such as treponematosis or degenerative conditions such as rheumatoid arthritis. Both of these infections are long-term, hence their opportunity to alter skeletal tissues, and only rarely would they have been the primary cause of death. Yet another shortcoming of skeletal analysis is the difficulty of identifying an infectious agent: in many cases, several conditions may affect bone tissue in the same way. For example, porotic hyperostosis, the porous enlargement of areas of the skull, can result from several circumstances, including anemia, scurvy, and infection.[11] In addition, lack of standardization in the identification and recording of bioarchaeological data hinders comparative analysis and further complicates the findings.[12]

But in spite of these problems, our understanding of health and mortality patterns in the New World before 1492 is expanding rapidly. And the profile that emerges resembles that of the Old World in several important respects: infant and child mortality was high and life expectancies low, and the primary causes of mortality were acute respiratory and gastrointestinal infections and periodic outbreaks of epidemic disease. In light of recent findings that reveal high levels of morbidity and mortality among pre-Columbian populations, it becomes increasingly difficult to argue that ancient Americans somehow managed to escape the scourge of epidemic disease so common in the rest of the world.

Nevertheless, significant differences existed between the disease environments of the Americas and the rest of the world, the most important being the absence of three specific crowd-type diseases: smallpox, measles, and bubonic plague. The origins of these particular infections will probably never be known, but if they existed among human populations in the Old World before waves of migration to the Americas began, they probably would not have survived the cold temperatures of the far north. And if they had, the low population levels of early hunter-gatherer societies would have precluded their permanent establishment in this hemisphere.

In addition, because of the absence of several species of quadrupeds, including cattle, horses, swine, goats, and sheep, native Americans domesticated fewer species of animals than did their contemporaries on other continents. Many Old World infections, including smallpox, measles, and plague, originated as zoonoses, diseases communicated from animals to humans under natural conditions, and although New World inhabitants eventually domesticated several species, including dogs, turkeys, ducks, and South American cameloids, smallpox, measles, bubonic plague, and cholera did not develop in the Americas.

Patterns of Mortality among Hunter-Gatherers

Between the period when humans first arrived in the western hemisphere some forty thousand years ago and the end of the fifteenth century, complex disease environments developed in response to specific regional conditions. Prior to the domestication of various food crops and the transition to sedentary, agricultural societies, a process that began in many areas between 7000 and 5000 BCE, human inhabitants of the Americas lived in small groups, migrating periodically in search of game and wild plant materials. At the end of the fifteenth century, the Arctic and Subarctic regions of Canada and Alaska, the Great Basin and southwestern areas of the United States, northern Mexico, the Amazon Basin, Patagonia, and Tierra del Fuego in southern South America all continued to support small hunter-gatherer populations. The nomadic and semisedentary peoples that lived in these challenging environments hunted, fished, gathered wild plants, and in some cases practiced forms of shifting agriculture.

The Arctic region, extending from northern Alaska across Canada, encompassed the harshest environment occupied by humans in the Americas. Little grew on the treeless tundra, where winters were long and dark and where the soil remained frozen year-round. Because of the challenges posed by this difficult place, permanent human settlement began here much later than it did in other areas. While waves of human immigrants passed through the Arctic region many thousands of years ago as they made their way east and south from Siberia, they did not remain here. The Inuits and Aleuts, who constituted the region's native population at the time of contact with Europeans, did not arrive until approximately 3000 BCE, when they came in boats from Siberia, Beringia having long ago submerged. As a result, these people were genetically distinct from other Amerindians, whose ancestors had arrived thousands of years earlier. Because of its remoteness and harsh climate, Europeans showed little interest in the Arctic region until the end of the eighteenth century.

Native inhabitants of the Arctic region all spoke languages related to one linguistic group, Eskimo-Aleut, providing further evidence of their common ancestry. Inuit and Aleut populations sustained themselves by hunting sea mammals and caribou and by fishing, but because of limited natural resources and the cold climate, their numbers always remained low.

Farther south, the climate of the Subarctic was somewhat more hospitable to human habitation than that of the far north, but winters in this area were still extremely harsh, and as a result, populations remained small. The Subarctic region spanned the North American continent from the Pacific coasts of southern Alaska and Canada to the Atlantic coast of Newfoundland, encompassing the interior of Alaska and most of Canada. Much of this area was covered by evergreen forests of pine, spruce, and fir. Many lakes, rivers, and streams also contributed to the distinctive environment of this region and provided early human populations with abundant supplies of fish and aquatic mammals. Small bands followed seasonal patterns of migration in search of food, hunting caribou, moose, musk ox, deer, beaver, otter, and mink. In addition, native populations supplemented their diet with fish and wild plants gathered during the short summer season. The native societies of this region, including the Koyukon, Chipewyan, Yellowknife, Cree, and Naskapi, all spoke languages related to two linguistic groups, Athapascan and Algonquian.

At the opposite end of the hemisphere, at the southern tip of South America, a cold climate also limited the size and complexity of human settlements. But while temperatures in Patagonia and Tierra del Fuego remained low year-round, this region was not as cold as the Arctic. At the end of the fifteenth century, dense forests covered the western slopes of the Andes, while grasslands predominated in the east, providing the human inhabitants of this area with abundant timber and wildlife resources. Nevertheless, because of the harshness of the environment and poor quality of the soils, human population levels were always low. A few native societies in this region engaged in slash-and-burn agriculture, a practice that involved felling and burning trees and undergrowth in order to clear land for temporary agricultural production, but most, including the Puelche and Tehuelche of Patagonia and the Ona and Haush of Tierra del Fuego, remained nomadic hunter-gatherers.

Just as cold temperatures in various regions of the Americas limited the growth of native populations, heat and a scarcity of water had similar effects. The harsh desert environment of the Great Basin, including the Death Valley region of California, covered a large area encompassing all of Utah and Nevada as well as parts of Colorado, Wyoming, Idaho, and

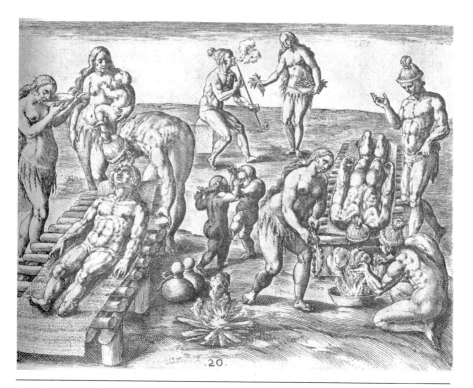

Fig. 8. *How the natives of Florida treat their sick. (Engraving by Theodore de Bry, 1591)*

Oregon. The basin itself was surrounded by the Rocky and Sierra Nevada Mountains, whose river systems drained into the basin. But because of scant precipitation, vegetation was sparse. As a result, the native peoples who inhabited this region were nomadic and survived by hunting small animals such as rabbits, birds, antelopes, and lizards and by gathering seeds, nuts, roots, and insects. This limited food supply checked population growth among scattered populations of Uto-Aztecan speakers, including the Ute, Paiute, and Shoshoni.

Similarly arid conditions prevailed in the southwestern part of what is today the United States and in northern Mexico, an area extending from southern Utah and Colorado through Arizona and New Mexico into the Mexican states of Chihuahua, Durango, Coahuila, and Tamaulipas. Plateaus, mountains, and desert dominated this region, which also included the eastern coast of the Gulf of California. Both agrarian and nomadic societies inhabited this area at the time of contact, but because of limited water resources, populations remained small. Agrarian societies included the Hopi, Zuni, Tewa, Keres, Tiwa, and Towa peoples, whose predecessors developed the most advanced agricultural practices north of central Mexico, including the use of extensive irrigation systems.

Nomadic peoples, including the Apache and Navajo, were Athapascan speakers from the north who arrived in the southwest between 800 and 1000 CE and who survived, in part, by raiding the settlements of agrarian populations. In fact, the Huichol, Guachichil, Concho, Pisones, and other nomadic peoples were regarded by residents of the highly developed Amerindian societies of central Mexico as *chichimecas*, or barbarians.

Archaeological research and studies of modern hunter-gatherer societies suggest that during the pre-Columbian period, a varied diet probably met the basic nutritional needs of most individuals, and as a result, illnesses related to nutritional deficiencies and malnutrition were rare. Famines occurred infrequently, but when they did, they were most likely to develop in areas with especially harsh climates such as the Arctic and Subarctic and in the driest regions of the southwestern United States and northern Mexico. While life expectancies at birth were short, they varied significantly from one society to another, from 16 to 22 years for males and 14 to 18 years for females, according to two samples.[13] This meant that few lived long enough to develop chronic, degenerative diseases associated with aging. Virtually everyone married young and polygamy was common, as was remarriage following the death of a spouse. Infant mortality rates were high—at least 40 percent of all children died by age 5. But because many women conceived soon after the death of an infant, birth rates also tended to be high. As might be expected, complications due to childbirth were a leading cause of death among women.[14] These demographic patterns among Amerindian populations closely resemble those of contemporaneous European and Asian populations.

Males, on the other hand, were more likely to sustain traumatic injuries either as a result of violence or accident.[15] Females also incurred trauma, but less frequently than males. Archaeological evidence reveals wide regional variation in the rate of traumatic injuries, but violent death resulting from "cannibalism, infanticide, sacrifice, geronticide, headhunting, and other forms of warfare" was common in many hunter-gatherer societies.[16] Skeletal remains from the southwestern United States reveal evidence of cannibalism, but whether it occurred in association with famine or war is unclear.[17] Mortality as a result of hunting accidents, exposure, and drowning occurred in many societies but was especially significant among inhabitants of the Arctic and Subarctic.[18]

Among the diseases common to hunter-gatherer populations, some, particularly bacterial and parasitic infections such as shigellosis, salmonellosis, tapeworms, hookworms, whipworms, and pinworms, accompanied human migrants directly from the Old World to the New and spread throughout the hemisphere. Both shigellosis and salmonellosis produce acute gastrointestinal illness, resulting in high morbidity and mortality especially among children, and both were found in the Americas prior to 1492. The former was most common in tropical areas, while the latter occurred more often among North American populations. While helminthic infections such as tapeworms, hookworms, whipworms, and pinworms did not pose a serious threat to public health, lack of energy and chronic malaise were common long-term side effects that reduced productivity and weakened the body's defenses against other infections.[19]

Because of their long association with the human species, two other groups of bacterial diseases, staphylococcal and streptococcal, also crossed the Bering Strait with immigrants to the Americas.[20] Both types of bacteria can cause illnesses ranging from minor skin and respiratory infections to potentially lethal conditions such as pneumonia, meningitis, and endocarditis. In their acute forms, staph and strep infections, especially pneumonia, would also have been leading causes of mortality in hunter-gatherer societies.[21]

Amebiasis, giardiasis, and toxoplasmosis, all protozoan infections, also undermined the health of early prehistoric populations in the Americas. Neither amebiasis nor giardiasis was in itself fatal, but during famines or in conjunction with other diseases their debilitating effects often contributed to higher mortality rates, especially among children. Toxoplasmosis was most serious when contracted during pregnancy because it could cause blindness, severe brain damage, or death of the fetus.

In addition to diseases arriving in the Americas with migrant populations, humans also encountered new diseases native to the hemisphere. New World leishmaniasis and American trypanosomiasis, or Chagas' disease, both transmitted by insect vectors, were protozoan infections especially prevalent in tropical areas. Another arthropod-transmitted illness was New World spotted fever. While this infection occurred throughout the hemisphere, it was especially common in North America, particularly west of the Rocky Mountains. Bartonellosis, or Carrion's disease, transmitted by sand flies, existed only in mountain valleys in northern South America. All of these infections were chronic and seldom fatal, but their presence could elevate mortality rates when other diseases or nutritional deficiencies developed.

Of the several spirochetal infections attacking pre-Hispanic populations, pinta, a nonvenereal treponematosis, was probably the most common in tropical areas. In temperate regions, especially eastern North America, another nonvenereal form of the disease was prevalent. Evidence of venereal treponematosis also exists, but so far it is limited to two cases, suggesting that this form of the disease was extremely rare.[22] In addition, three other spirochetal diseases, leptospirosis and two types of relapsing fever, were also native to the Americas. Leptospirosis, transmitted through contaminated water, soil, and food, was rarely fatal, but occasionally complications such as anemia, meningitis, or hemorrhaging developed. Endemic relapsing fever, transmitted by ticks, was less severe than the louse-borne epidemic variety, which could produce mortality rates of up to 50 percent.

Acute respiratory infections, especially pneumonia, a frequent cause of death in the period following the development of sedentary, agricultural societies, were also the major cause of mortality among hunter-gatherer populations throughout the hemisphere.[23] Archaeological evidence suggests that tuberculosis has a long history among human inhabitants of the New World: the earliest remains showing clear signs of the disease date back some two thousand years.[24] But according to one author, among small, nomadic populations of the early prehistoric period, the disease could not have been sustained for long periods because it would have posed a serious threat to the continued survival of the group; therefore it probably occurred infrequently.[25] Two other respiratory infections, blastomycosis and coccidioidomycosis, both caused by fungi transmitted in soil, were uncommon among nonagricultural peoples.

In large part, demographic factors determined patterns of mortality in hunter-gatherer societies. Small, mobile populations seldom experienced outbreaks of epidemic disease, but because most individuals in these populations were always under the age of twenty, infections of childhood were especially common. Respiratory and gastrointestinal illnesses, including pneumonia, tuberculosis, shigellosis, salmonellosis, amebiasis, and giardiasis, were the leading causes of mortality among all age groups, but they struck particularly hard at infants and children under the age of five. Other infections such as leishmaniasis, trypanosomiasis, leptospirosis, and relapsing fever had a greater impact on the health of adults, whose daily tasks placed them in more frequent contact with the insect vectors that transmitted these diseases.[26] Among women, complications arising from childbirth were a leading cause of death throughout the hemisphere. The frequency of death due to traumatic injuries from social violence or accidents varied significantly from one region to another, but in some areas, violent trauma claimed the lives of many, especially postadolescent males. For example, 16 percent of the skeletons recovered at a site in the Illinois River Valley show signs of trauma and violent death, including projectile points embedded in the remains, unhealed fractures, and scalping.[27] At one site occupied by the Pueblos of the southwestern United States, the frequency of traumatic injury reached 41 percent, and skeletal remains revealed evidence of massacres and cannibalism.[28]

Patterns of Mortality among Sedentary Agriculturalists

Although climate and resources limited the growth of population in specific areas of the Americas, vast expanses of territory proved far more hospitable to social development. In these regions, the number of inhabitants increased, supported by intensive farming practices and the development of agricultural technologies appropriate to specific environments. At the end of the fifteenth century, villages and towns dotted the landscapes of the northwest Pacific coast, California, the Columbia Plateau, the Great Plains, the north and southeastern Atlantic coastline of the United States, the islands of the Caribbean, southern Central America, northern South America, and the Atlantic coast of South America. Small elites dominated these societies, with chiefs distributing resources, assigning labor obligations, and mediating social disputes. These chiefdoms represent an intermediate level of social development among Amerindian societies, a level between nomadic hunter-gatherers and the more highly structured state systems of the Mexica and Incas.

The northwest coastal area stretched from northern California into western Oregon, Washington, and British Columbia, terminating in southern Alaska. The terrain was rugged, dominated by the Cascade Mountains and bordered on the west by many inlets and islands. As a result of the moist, mild climate and abundant natural resources, this region supported a large native population at the time of contact. Unlike other regions of the Americas, where human populations expanded in response to agricultural increase, in the northwest, generous supplies of fish and game enabled natives to establish permanent villages while adopting labor-intensive agricultural practices only for the production of such nonessentials as tobacco. In fact, the natural wealth of the region supported the development of complex societies, where individuals vied for prestige by giving away material commodities, a practice known as potlatch. Many societies inhabited the northwest coastal region, including Na-Dene speakers such as the Tlingit, Haida, and Eyak, as well as those who spoke Penutian languages, including the Chinook, Coos, and Tsimshians.

Owing to an abundance of natural resources, the native population of California and Baja California in present-day Mexico was the densest in North America at the time of contact. As was the case in the Pacific Northwest, nature's bounty precluded the necessity of agricultural production: the region's mild climate, extensive coastline, and northern river systems provided humans with a varied diet, including fish, shellfish, deer, small game, acorns, and other wild plants. The area's large native population, composed of many ethnic and linguistic groups, including the Shasta, Salina, Maidu, Cahuilla, Kiliwa, and Chumash, had settled in permanent villages along the coast and in river valleys.

The Columbia Plateau occupied an area encompassing eastern Washington, northern Idaho, western Montana, northeast and central Oregon, and southeast British Columbia. The environment of this region varied widely from the Cascade and Rocky Mountain chains in the west and east, to desert in the south, to cold forest and hills in the north. Amerindian villages, many of them situated along the banks of the Columbia, Fraser, and Snake Rivers, harvested much of their food, especially salmon, trout, and sturgeon, from the waters. In addition, rivers provided transportation for both people and their commodities. Although not as densely settled as those of the northwest, native populations, including the Nez Perce, Chinook, Spokane, and Flathead, had developed complex societies governed by political chiefs.

The Great Plains extended from the Mississippi River in the east to the Rocky Mountains in the west and from southern Canada in the north to southern Texas. Before the arrival of Europeans, the largely treeless grasslands of this region provided grazing range for huge herds of bison. Following the introduction of the horse to the Great Plains, many Amerindian societies adopted a nomadic way of life, but prior to the sixteenth century, these native populations lived in villages, often situated in river valleys, and depended more on agriculture. Among the earliest inhabitants of this region were Siouan speakers, including the Mandans, Witchita, and Pawnee, and later arrivals such as the Cheyenne, Cree, Ojibway, Crow, Sioux, and Apache.

Amerindian populations of the northeast inhabited an area extending from the Atlantic coast across the Appalachians to the Mississippi Valley and from the Great Lakes to the Tidewater region of Virginia and North Carolina. At the beginning of the sixteenth century, deciduous and coniferous forests covered much of this vast area, providing wood for the construction of shelters and the manufacture of tools as well as habitat for the many species of animals on which indigenous populations depended for food. Many ethnic groups, both hunter-gatherers and agriculturists, occupied the region at the time of contact. Archaeologists and anthropologists have divided these societies into five linguistic groups: the Nova Scotia, New England, Long Island, Hudson Valley, and Delaware Valley Algonquian speakers, including the Micmac, Massachuset, Narraganset, Mahican, and Delaware tribes; the New York and Ontario Iroquoian speakers, including the Mohawk, Oneida, Seneca, Erie, and Huron; the Great Lakes Algonquians, including the Ottawa, Menominee, and some Ojibway; the Prairie Algonquians, including the Fox, Kickapoo, Miami, and Shawnee; and the southern-fringe societies, both Algonquian and Iroquoian speaking, including the Powhatan, Nanticoke, Tuscarora, and Seotan.

The southeast culture area extended from the Atlantic Ocean into Texas and from the Gulf of Mexico into Oklahoma, Arkansas, Missouri, Kentucky, West Virginia, Maryland, Virginia, and North Carolina. The climate here was generally mild, especially along the coastal plain and marshes of the east and south; mountainous regions in the west had longer, colder winters. Like the northeast, this area was heavily forested at the beginning of the sixteenth century. The majority of native societies organized themselves around agricultural production, but some groups were nonagriculturists, sustaining themselves through hunting, gathering, and fishing. Agrarian peoples lived in villages, moving periodically as soils became depleted. Languages from many linguistic groups, including Muskogean, Siouan, Iroquoian, and Algonquian, were spoken in this region. The southeast was home to the Cherokee, Choctaw, Chickasaw, Creek, and Seminole, as well as others such as the Catawba, Alabamba, and Natchez.

Scholars have described the Circum-Caribbean, extending from southern El Salvador and Honduras through Central America, across the Isthmus of Panama, and into northern South America, as a geographical, biological, and cultural bridge between North and South America. And in fact, the human societies of this region shared much in common. The mountain chains that dominated the landscapes of Mexico and Guatemala continued, albeit somewhat diminished, through Central America, rising once again in northern South America to become the towering mountains of the Andes. Narrow coastal plains bordered the region along its Pacific and Caribbean rims as far as southern Panama; in northern Colombia and Venezuela, a wide floodplain spread out along the Caribbean coast. Except for the Guajira Peninsula of Colombia, which was extremely arid most of the year, the rest of the region received heavy rainfall, and parts of southern Panama were so wet that agriculture was almost impossible.

Archaeological evidence suggests that humans first passed through this area at least twenty thousand years ago. During the Archaic period (7000–2000 BCE), humans established permanent communities based on agricultural production and fishing. Each community was controlled by a chief, and powerful leaders governed at the regional level. These societies developed technological advances in ceramic production and metallurgy, and they engaged in long-distance trade in gold and other luxury commodities with societies in Mexico, northern Central America, and the Andes. The native populations of this region, including the Tairona, Muisca, Sinu, and Cuna, spoke languages related to a single linguistic group, Macro-Chibchan.

When Europeans arrived in the Caribbean at the end of the fifteenth century, tropical forests covered most of the islands of the Greater and Lesser Antilles. Human settlement of the region had begun thousands of years before, when nonhorticultural peoples from the eastern coast of Central America colonized the islands. Then, sometime around 200 to 300 BCE, another group of migrants from the northeastern coast of Venezuela set out in canoes to fish the coral reefs and mangroves of neighboring islands. Beginning on the island of Trinidad and slowly moving north over the course of many generations, these people occupied the entire region. At the time of contact with Europeans, dense populations of Arawak-speaking Indians dominated the Caribbean, having conquered the hunter-gatherer societies that preceded them. The Arawaks were farmers, cultivating maize, manioc, beans, and squash, all introduced from the mainland, as well as hunter-gatherers. The highest developments in Arawak culture, known as Taino, occurred on the islands of Hispaniola, Puerto Rico, and Cuba. Taino society was organized into chiefdoms comprising numerous villages, some of them quite large. Not long before the Spanish arrived in the Americas, another wave of migrants from northeastern South America began to challenge Arawak control of the Lesser Antilles. The Caribs were a warrior society, less developed than their rivals, and it was the Caribs who resisted European conquest of the Caribbean most fiercely.

The Atlantic coast of South America, from the Guianas to southern Brazil, was the home to large populations of culturally diverse peoples at the time of contact. While the topography of this vast region varies from flatlands in the north to the hills and cliffs of the south, most of the area was covered in dense forests. In response to this tropical environment, human populations adopted two patterns of settlement: hunting, gathering, and fishing; and slash-and-burn agriculture. But because of the poor nature of tropical soils, villages relocated every few years. When the Portuguese arrived on the coast of Brazil in 1500, they encountered large stockaded villages of Tupi speakers, living communally in longhouses containing thirty or more families.

In the vast lowlands of Amazonia, stretching from eastern Colombia, Ecuador, Peru, and Bolivia into western Venezuela, the Guianas, and Brazil, heavy rainfall, high temperatures, and poor soils combined to limit the size of human populations; nevertheless, at least by the sixteenth century, some regions supported large indigenous communities. The Amazon River system was composed of many tributaries, creating a vast floodplain. Much of this area was covered in dense tropical forests, teeming with thousands of species of flora and fauna. Archaeological

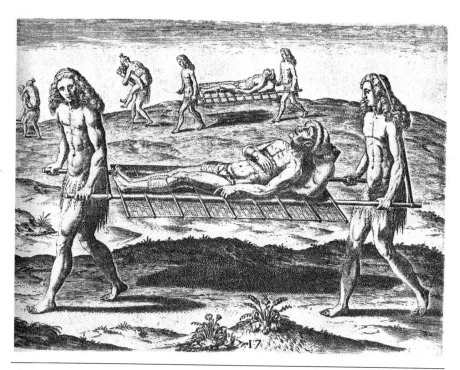

Fig. 9.   *Florida natives transport the sick and the dead. (Engraving by Theodore de Bry, 1591)*

evidence indicates that humans arrived in Amazonia at least ten thousand years ago and went on to develop two subsistence patterns, hunting and gathering and slash-and-burn farming. When Europeans began exploring Amazonia during the sixteenth century, they encountered societies that spoke many languages, including Arawak and Carib, languages most often associated with Caribbean peoples, suggesting that this region had long been a crossroads for many different cultures.

Of the many regions of the Americas conducive to human settlement and cultural development, two locations stand out from all the rest. Before 1492, the largest populations and most highly developed state systems in the New World evolved in Mesoamerica and the Andean highlands. Hierarchical class structures, divisions of labor, and occupational specialization all characterized the societies of the Mexica, Mayas, and Incas. In order to support dense populations, each group had adapted technologies specific to the environments in which they lived. Large-scale agricultural economies generated wealth sufficient to support elites as well as the development of extensive trade networks and professional merchant classes.

Mesoamerica is the term applied to the cultural area that extends from central Mexico to northern Central America. Mountain ranges dominated the landscape, bordered on each side by the narrow coastal plains of the Gulf of Mexico and the Pacific Ocean. To the east lay the Yucatán Peninsula, a limestone platform jutting out into the Gulf of Mexico. The entire Mesoamerican region lay within tropical latitudes, but climatic conditions varied significantly depending on altitude. Highland areas that became the focus of dense human settlement were characterized by moderate temperatures and scant rainfall, making the use of irrigation for agricultural production a necessity. Lowland populations, on the other hand, lived in a warm, moist environment that required the development of distinctly different agricultural techniques, including systems for draining wetlands.

Archaeologists have found evidence of human settlement in Mesoamerica dating back at least fifteen thousand years. The archaeological record also reveals that humans began the domestication of maize and other food plants in this region sometime around 7000 BCE. By 2000 BCE, advanced agricultural techniques and ceramic production were well established, and much of the human population was living in villages controlled by chiefs. At the end of the fifteenth century, the Mexica controlled most of central and southern Mexico, while Maya city-states dominated Yucatán and northern Central America. Both the Mexica and Mayas had inherited their cultural traditions from the many societies that had preceded them in their respective territories. Both societies were highly stratified with powerful elite classes dominating political, religious, and economic activities. Technically sophisticated agricultural systems fed dense urban populations. Long-distance trade and transportation networks supported diverse economies that produced a variety of material artifacts, including different types of cloth, jewelry, ceramics, and featherwork. Like their predecessors, Mexica and Maya elites drafted large numbers of laborers for public works projects, including the construction of monumental stone buildings, many of which remain standing today. Even Spaniards who had traveled widely throughout Europe and the Middle East were impressed by the size, beauty, and complexity of Mesoamerican cities.

Farther south in the Andes, parallel chains of mountains dominated the landscape of the area extending from Colombia south through Ecuador and into Peru and Bolivia. The terrain was extremely rugged, encompassing a series of microclimates that changed with altitudinal variations. A narrow coastal plain bordered the region along the Pacific coast. Life for humans in this region was difficult owing to the dry conditions that prevailed along the coastline and the high altitudes, cold, and aridity that characterized life in the highlands. In addition, beneath the long, narrow valleys flanked by towering volcanoes lay a series of geological faults, the periodic shifting of which produced violent earthquakes and volcanic eruptions.

To date, the earliest evidence of human occupation of this region stretches back some ten thousand years. By 3000 BCE, a series of native societies along the coast of Peru were living in large, urban communities, constructing stepped pyramids, some as high as ten stories. This development coincided with the building of the pyramids in Egypt and preceded similar developments in Mesoamerica by a thousand years. By 2000 BCE, complex societies had also developed in the highlands. At the time of contact, the Inca state dominated an area extending from southern Colombia to northern Chile and from the Pacific coast into the Amazon Basin. Like that of the Mexica, Inca society was built upon the foundations established by the many cultures that had preceded it. Inca society was also highly stratified, governed by a powerful elite ruling from their administrative capital in the city of Cuzco, situated in the southern highlands of Peru. The Incas and their predecessors relied on sophisticated agricultural techniques, including complex irrigation networks and terracing, to produce enough food to feed large populations. An extensive network of roads and bridges, linking large-scale storage facilities and way stations, facilitated long-distance trade and travel throughout the region.

The demographic increase of human populations throughout the Americas following the domestication of food crops and the widespread adoption of agriculture practices altered patterns of mortality in significant ways. While all of the threats to health and life prevalent in hunter-gatherer societies continued to exist, new problems developed as the result of dietary changes and increasingly dense populations. According to archaeologists and paleopathologists, the transition to a sedentary, agricultural way of life had a negative impact on the health of human populations around the world. A largely vegetarian diet, often composed almost entirely of one or two food crops, replaced the varied, more nutritionally balanced diet of hunter-gatherers.

In many regions of the Americas, corn, deficient in several key nutrients, became the dietary staple of agriculturalists, and as a result, health problems related to nutritional deficiencies increased significantly in most, but not all, sedentary societies.[29] One very visible indication of declining dietary standards among Mesoamerican populations is a temporal and regional decline in human stature occurring on a north-south axis: the skeletal remains of northerners, who adopted agricultural practices later and continued to consume a more varied diet, with higher levels of animal protein, displayed greater mean heights than those of southerners, who earlier adopted a corn-based diet.[30] A similar decline in stature occurred among prehistoric residents of coastal Georgia following their transition to sedentary agricultural settlements.[31]

Shorter stature is only one indicator of declining health among New World agriculturalists. Throughout the Americas, archaeologists and paleopathologists have uncovered a pattern of rising rates of undernutrition, decreased resistance, and increased frequency of infection. A high incidence of porotic hyperostosis, dental caries, and Harris lines, especially among young children, ages two to four, suggests that mothers often weaned their offspring on a corn pap, leading, in many instances, to protein-energy malnutrition. This condition, in combination with parasitic or other infections, often precipitated a crisis, resulting in the death of the child.[32] Owing to the physiological stress of weaning and the possible impairment of their immunological systems, many who survived continued to experience high rates of infection throughout their often short lives.[33] Because corn is deficient in iron and niacin, the incidence of anemia and pellagra increased. In many societies, anemia was common in individuals of both sexes and all age groups, but especially so among pregnant women and children, both of whom required larger amounts of iron than other segments of the population. In populations heavily dependent on corn, iron-deficiency anemia became a serious problem throughout the Americas, particularly in tropical areas, where chronic parasitic infections further increased iron losses.[34]

Like their human counterparts in the Old World, sedentary populations throughout the Americas expanded in spite of poor nutrition and rising rates of infection. This increase, in the face of declining health, was due to several factors. First, the availability of corn pap allowed mothers to wean their children at an earlier age, thus decreasing the time between birth intervals. This allowed women to bear more children over the course of their reproductive lives. One scholar has calculated that in prehistoric Mexico, females who survived to puberty could expect to bear a child every 3 to 4 years. Thus a woman who lived to menopause, though few did, might produce eight or more offspring.[35] So while mortality rates increased in agricultural societies, so did fertility rates. In addition, while several studies suggest that agriculturalists lived slightly longer lives (by approximately 2 to 4 years) than did hunter-gatherers, others indicate a decline.[36] Human remains from sites in northern Chile and northern Peru also indicate that at least in some societies, members of the elite enjoyed better health, though not necessarily longer lives, than the rest of the population.[37] But data from Teotihuacan in Mexico reveal that during periods of stress associated with population pressure, shrinking food supplies, and social strife, life expectancies at birth actually declined significantly, from 24 years during the early Classic (200–400 CE) to 16 years during the late Classic (650–750 CE) period.[38] Calculations of average life expectancy in various regions of the Old World show similar fluctuations. For example, studies indicate that in classical Greece, the mean age at death was 27 to 30, while the average life expectancy at birth in imperial Rome ranged over time from a low of 15 to a high of 25. During the Middle Ages, average life expectancies in Europe rose to a high of 30 years during the period between 750 and 1000 CE.[39] But on average, people in the Old World before 1500 probably lived between 20 and 25 years.

Thus, while it remains unclear whether or not agricultural peoples lived slightly longer or shorter lives than did hunter-gatherers, life expectancies of people in the pre-Columbian Americas were probably comparable to those of their counterparts in western Europe. Certainly no evidence exists to support Guaman Poma's claim that before the arrival of Europeans, native peoples lived long and healthy lives.

With the transition to sedentary agricultural communities and the accompanying demographic expansion came increased social contact and increased frequency of infection. Diseases associated with crowding and poor sanitation became common, and when they developed in individuals already weakened by undernutrition and parasitic infections, they often proved fatal. Gastrointestinal infections such as amebiasis, giardiasis, and salmonellosis, long prevalent among hunter-gatherer populations, flourished in the often contaminated water and food supplies of village dwellers and continued to claim many lives, especially among the young. Over time, as agricultural populations increased, so too did the degree of urbanization, and with increased population density came significantly higher rates of gastrointestinal infections. While the prevalence of treponematoses, especially pinta and yaws, increased as a result of expanded social contacts, these infections remained chronic and seldom fatal.

But agriculturalists also contended with diseases seldom experienced by hunter-gatherers and even some illnesses previously unknown. Acute respiratory infections continued to pose the greatest threat to the lives of native Americans, and within densely settled regions, tuberculosis appeared with increasing frequency. The tuberculosis bacilli, inhaled or ingested in contaminated food, could affect any organ of the body, but in the Americas, the pulmonary and spinal forms of the disease were most common. In its chronic, pulmonary form, individuals experienced fatigue, fever, weight loss, and coughing. Skeletal remains from North America indicate that the disease was so common that "virtually every member of these late prehistoric communities had primary exposure to tuberculosis."[40] A similar situation probably prevailed in highland areas of Mesoamerica and the Andes. This infection was especially lethal in children and young adults, but in conjunction with other illnesses, malnutrition, and crowded, unsanitary conditions, mortality increased among all segments of the population.

Tissue samples also indicate that bacterial pneumonia was common and that many individuals contracted the disease more than once.[41] When pneumonia appeared in association with tuberculosis and other diseases, death often followed. Yet another serious, though much less common, respiratory infection was blastomycosis. Although the fungus responsible for producing the disease lived in soils throughout the hemisphere, it occurred more often in tropical and subtropical regions of South America, where those engaged in agricultural activities were most susceptible. The fungus produced lesions on the lungs, mucous membranes, and skin and frequently resulted in death.

One can also build a strong case for the existence of both endemic (flea-borne) and epidemic (louse-borne) typhus in the New World before 1492. In both tropical and temperate zones, rodents and other small mammals, often living in close proximity to humans, served as reservoirs for the endemic form of the disease. Historian Hans Zinsser speculates that isolated cases of endemic typhus probably occurred long before the illness developed into its epidemic form.[42] Thus while some hunter-gatherer populations probably experienced the endemic illness, epidemic typhus was a new disease that appeared in association with crowded, unsanitary conditions. Human remains reveal that head and body lice commonly infested sedentary populations. Lice prefer cool climates, and the heavy woolen and cotton clothing worn by residents of temperate regions of North America, Mesoamerica, and the Andes provided safe habitats for these parasites. Epidemic typhus was transmitted directly from one human to another by the bite of an infected body louse. Both forms of the disease began suddenly with fever, chills, severe headaches, exhaustion, and general pain. A skin eruption appeared by the fifth or sixth day, often accompanied by delirium and deafness. Death resulted from a collapse of the cardiovascular system. During the twentieth century, mortality rates for endemic typhus averaged 2 percent and climbed to 10 to 40 percent for the epidemic variety.

Preconquest traditions of epidemics occurring during periods of social turmoil—wars, famines, and natural disasters—support the assertion that typhus may have existed in the Americas before the sixteenth century. In his history of the Incas, Guaman Poma described two epidemics that occurred before the Spanish conquest. In recounting the military achievements of Pachacuti Inca Yupanqui (1438–1471), Guaman Poma wrote:

> The defeat of Chile was made possible by the ravages of plague, which lasted for ten years. Disease and famine, even more than force of arms, brought about the downfall of the Chileans, just as civil war between Huascar and Atahualpa was later to facilitate the Spanish conquest. Peru itself suffered terribly from plague, famine, and drought. For a decade no rain fell and the grass withered and died. People were reduced to devouring their own children and when the stomachs of the poor were opened it was sometimes found that they had managed to survive by eating grasses.[43]

Furthermore, Guaman Poma wrote that the Incas associated "a plague of fleas" with death, suggesting that they may have connected these ectoparasites with the appearance of typhus.[44]

In pre-Columbian Mesoamerica, a similar association developed between famines and outbreaks of epidemic disease. Both Mexica and Maya historical accounts contain references to periods of disease related to natural disasters and famines.[45] Although some historians argue that typhus was not present in Mexico before contact, others claim that it was.[46] Certainly the dense populations of highland Mesoamerica would have provided an attractive habitat for typhus rickettsiae. In 1576, an epidemic often diagnosed as typhus broke out in central Mexico; the Mexica called the disease *matlazahuatl*, meaning eruptions that appeared on the skin in a regular netlike pattern, suggesting that they were already familiar with the illness.[47] Furthermore, one historian claims that the representation of an individual covered with the skin eruptions characteristic of typhus was included in a pre-Columbian codex.[48]

According to historian Sherburne F. Cook, the Mexica recounted five periods of epidemic disease in their preconquest history. All of the descriptions are vague, but one outbreak that occurred at the end of the late thirteenth century involved an inflammation of the skin, which Cook translated as "splitting or cracking of all the flesh."[49] While this pathology could have been caused by any number of diseases, epidemic typhus is a possibility. Mexica history also recorded a period of significant mortality that occurred during the 1450s. Pre-Columbian traditions recount a cycle of natural disaster, famine, disease, and death beginning with a freezing winter that occurred either in 1450–1451 or 1453–1454. A three-year drought followed, resulting in mass famine and the appearance of disease. Descriptions differ, but one source noted the presence of "pestilencial catarrh," another "fuego," a possible reference to fever, skin eruptions, or rash. Cook argues that no evidence indicates any diseases other than those resulting directly from malnutrition and starvation were present; on the other hand, it is possible that typhus, or some other serious epidemic disease, was circulating among the already weakened population.[50]

It also seems likely that typhus may have existed in temperate regions of North America during the late prehistoric period. Among the precontact Ontario Iroquoians the presence of refuse dumps, scavenging animals, crowded, longhouse living conditions, and migrants from other societies provided an environment conducive to the spread of epidemic diseases, including fevers, encephalitides, rabies, typhus, dysentery, pneumonia, and tuberculosis.[51] If that was indeed the case, then typhus probably ravaged other agricultural societies in temperate regions of North America, and, in fact, increased contact between various native societies during the late prehistoric period could easily have facilitated the spread of the disease from one settlement to another. But because typhus does not leave physical markers, we may never know for certain whether or not it existed in the New World before 1492. If it did, typhus would have been one of the most lethal of all diseases and a significant cause of mortality.

Similarly, scholars have uncovered no data regarding the existence of influenza in pre-Columbian America, but circumstantial evidence suggests that this disease also may have appeared by the late prehistoric period, if not earlier in some areas. Viral influenza infects many animals, including humans, pigs, and fowl. Recent studies indicate that influenza viruses originating among populations of domesticated ducks are responsible for the most lethal outbreaks, and, as already stated, ducks were among the species domesticated by prehistoric Americans.[52] Crosby speculates that influenza probably appeared in many regions of the world with the development of agriculture and the domestication of animals.[53] Others have also suggested that influenza may have been present in densely populated regions of the Americas long before the arrival of Europeans.[54] In his study of pandemic influenza, Patterson posits that wild ducks or other migratory birds could have introduced the virus to New World duck populations, leading to its eventual transfer to humans. He also explains that because of the virus's ability to mutate rapidly and its antigenic variability, "the disease can maintain itself in much smaller populations than, for example, measles or smallpox."[55] Influenza was characterized by its abrupt onset signaled by fever, chills, headache, sore throat, and cough. Epidemics developed and spread rapidly, often appearing in temperate zones during the winter. In tropical regions, timing was not related to seasons. Complications, including pneumonia, often developed, escalating mortality rates, especially among the elderly and young adults. Influenza could have been responsible for the "pestilencial catarrh" and "fuego" (in this case "fuego" would be translated as fever) that the Mexica described in association with the famine and epidemic of 1454–1457.

It should come as no surprise to note that among sedentary populations, depending as they did on agricultural production for their continued survival, malnutrition and famines occurred with greater regularity than they did among hunter-gatherers. As previously mentioned, the histories of the Incas, Mexica, and Mayas all contain accounts of prolonged droughts followed by periods of famine and disease. The Maya *Book of Chilam Balam* includes several references to drought and famine during the prehistoric period.[56] One of these occurred during Katun 4 Ahua (1480–1485):

> The face of the lord of the katun is covered; his face is dead. There is mourning for water; there is mourning for bread. His mat and his throne shall face the west. Blood-vomit is the charge of the katun.[57]

Insufficient information prohibits a reliable diagnosis, but one author speculates that this may be the same outbreak described years later by Bishop Landa. In that case, the symptoms included fever, body swelling, and infestations of "worms."[58] Bloody vomit could have resulted from acute gastroenteritis; "worms" could be a reference to intestinal parasites or to the larvae of flies or other insects that laid their eggs in festering sores.

Inca history recounts the harrowing episode of the ten-year-long drought and famine that reduced some people to eating their own children. *The Huarochiri Manuscript,* a compilation of Andean traditions recorded during the early seventeenth century, also includes references to famine and periods of overpopulation.[59] Among the Mexica, memories of hunger and death lingered long; traditions recall famines that occurred around 1330, between 1454 and 1457, and again between 1504 and 1506.[60] Both gastrointestinal and respiratory infections accompanied the famine of 1330, resulting in many deaths.[61] Famines could also be exacerbated or manipulated for political and economic purposes. For example, during the drought and famine in parts of central Mexico between 1454 and 1457, the coastal-dwelling Totonacs of Vera Cruz, longtime enemies of the Mexica, exploited the situation by trading food for slaves. According to one account:

> They [the Totonacs] came to Tenochtitlán carrying great loads of maize in order to buy slaves. They also went to other cities— Tezcoco, Chalco, Xochimilco, and the Tepanec center, Tacuba— where they purchased large numbers of slaves with their corn. They placed yokes around the necks of adults and children. Then the slaves, lined up one behind another, were led out of the cities in a pitiful manner, the husband leaving his wife, the father his son, the grandmother her grandchild. They went along weeping and their wails reached the heavens. In this way a great number of people from all these nations became slaves. Others without having been sold went freely to the land of the Totonacs with their wives and children, where they settled permanently and where they remain to this day. Others, in their desire to escape the province, fell dead along the way, together with the loads they carried.[62]

Undoubtedly, these fragments describe only a few of the famines that occurred in the pre-Columbian Americas. Owing to the destruction of preconquest records, the disruption and loss of many oral traditions, and the fallibility of human memory, evidence regarding other natural disasters, famines, and epidemics has been lost forever.

Archaeological evidence also indicates that levels of violence increased among agricultural populations.[63] Competition for resources in densely populated areas often resulted in violence between individuals and entire societies. The Mexica, Incas, Mayas, and their predecessors all waged massive military campaigns against neighboring populations in order to expand their territorial control over human labor and natural resources. At various times during the precontact period, mortality as a result of interpersonal or intersocietal violence was significant. For example, the Incas were forced to mount four costly campaigns in order to conquer the rebellious Carangues and Cayambes of northern Ecuador. Following the final battle, around 1500, Inca soldiers carried out a massacre on the shores of Lake Yaguarcocha. According to the Spanish chronicler, Pedro Cieza de León, more than 20,000 adult males from the Otavalo area died in this battle.[64] The Inca army staged another massacre in southern Ecuador shortly before the arrival of Francisco Pizarro; in this case, the army of Atahualpa Inca slew "more than 35,000 Canari males and left many wounded."[65] Another Spaniard describing the same incident wrote, "Of 50,000 not more than 3,000 remained."[66] Mexica and Maya armies also engaged in major military confrontations, often claiming thousands of lives.

While the native populations of North America were not as large as those of Mesoamerica and the Andes, by the late prehistoric period, skeletal evidence indicates high rates of mortality related to violence in many areas. At one site in the central Illinois River valley, one-third of all adults died as a result of violent injuries. Similar patterns of violence appear at sites in northwestern Alabama, the northern Great Plains, northern California, and Michigan. Evidence of scalping is especially common; at the Crow Creek site in the Missouri River valley, 90 percent of all crania showed signs of scalping. Decapitation as well as nose and tongue removal also occurred. Human remains indicate that adult males died as a result of violence more often than females, but at one site in Michigan, archaeologists have found a significantly higher rate of fatal injuries in adult women between the ages of twenty-one and twenty-five than in males. Spousal abuse or bride raiding have been suggested as possible explanations for this anomaly.[67]

The preceding analysis of mortality among ancient Americans dispels the long-cherished myth of a pre-Columbian paradise. Like their Old World counterparts, before 1492, residents of the New World died as a result of disease, famine, and violence. While the disease environment of the Americas may have differed from that of the Old World in terms of particular diseases, the leading causes of mortality among humans in all parts of the world were basically the same—acute respiratory and gastrointestinal infections. Residents of the Old World were exposed to a wider variety of epidemic diseases, but typhus and influenza may have been universal among agricultural populations. Similarly, periodic famines, attended by high rates of mortality, were a regular occurrence for agricultural populations around the world. And certainly there is ample evidence to suggest that native Americans were just as violent as their counterparts in other regions of the globe. But in spite of disease patterns that were strikingly similar in some important respects, native Americans were not immunologically prepared for the devastation that lay ahead.

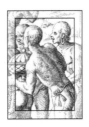

3 • Colonialism, Disease, and the Spanish Conquest of the Caribbean, Mesoamerica, and the Central Andes

*I*t is hopeless to speak of its natives, because forty years have already elapsed since the conquest of the island [Hispaniola], and . . . almost all are gone. Of five hundred thousand inhabitants of various nations and languages that existed on the island forty years ago, there remain fewer than twenty thousand living; a large number died from the smallpox, others perished in the wars, still others in the gold mines where Christians forced them to work against their nature, because they are weak people, and poor workers.

Nicolas Federmann, *Viaje a las Indians del Mar Oceano*

It is said that in the past there were many more Indians, and so it seems from the lay of the land. . . . The Indians have diminished with the wars that they fought against the Incas and later with the conquest by the Spanish and finally with certain epidemics of smallpox and measles and typhus that have occurred in this area; and with these things they have been reduced.

Juan Sancho Paz Ponce de León,
"Relacion y descripción de los pueblos del partido de Otavalo"

The Introduction of Old World Diseases to the Americas

Europeans who came to colonize the New World left their homelands for a variety of reasons. Some sought wealth and personal glory, others political and religious freedom. But whatever their individual motivations, driving the movement of people from the Old World to the New was a rapidly expanding European economic system, fueled by demographic growth, increased trade, and technological advancements such as the mariner's compass and improvements in ship design. For centuries, many in Europe sought to circumvent the monopoly that Venetian and Egyptian merchants had established over the lucrative eastern Mediterranean trade for Asian spices, silks, and other valuable commodities. Following the capture of the Moroccan port of Ceuta in 1415, Portugal assumed the lead in the search for an alternate route to the Far East. Under the sponsorship of Prince Henry, "the Navigator" (1394–1460), and later King John II (1481–1495), Portuguese sailors gradually extended their explorations down the western coast of Africa, rounding the Cape of Good Hope in 1487. A decade later, the Portuguese nobleman Vasco da Gama reached India, and in 1500, Pedro Alvares Cabral, also on his way to India, accidentally landed on the coast of Brazil.

Ferdinand of Aragon and Isabelle of Castile also coveted a share of the Asian trade and, when the defeat of Moslem forces at Granada appeared imminent in the early 1490s, they agreed to support the expedition of a Genoese sailor, Christopher Columbus. After a ten-week voyage across the Atlantic, Columbus and his crew landed in the Bahama Islands in October 1492. While Columbus continued to assert that he had indeed reached Asia, Isabella and her advisers moved quickly to consolidate Castilian control over what they realized was previously unclaimed territory. In 1494, Isabella signed the Treaty of Tordesillas, establishing the boundary between Spanish and Portuguese claims in the Americas. That demarcation, running some 370 leagues west of the Azores, limited Portuguese colonization to Brazil and ceded all territory west of the line to Castile. Despite this treaty the boundary between Brazil and Spanish territories was disputed, often violently, until the last decades of the eighteenth century.

The initial focus of Spanish conquest and settlement was the islands of the Caribbean and the eastern coast of Central America. Except for establishing a limited number of settlements along the coast, the Portuguese ignored the colonization of Brazil for many years, focusing instead on their richer Asian and African possessions. Following the conquest of the Caribbean and parts of Central America, the Spanish attempted to extend their control to other regions, sending expeditions into North America in 1513 and then again in the 1520s and 1540s.

By the early 1520s, Spanish troops led by Hernán Cortés and aided by thousands of Indian allies and an epidemic of smallpox, controlled much of Mexico and northern Central America. Similarly, by 1540, Spaniards ruled large sections of the former Inca empire, which encompassed an area from southern Colombia through Ecuador, Peru, and Bolivia into northern Chile. From this base in the Andes, Europeans fanned out in all directions, establishing settlements throughout northern South America and the Amazon Basin. With the permanent founding of Buenos Aires in 1580, Spain effectively controlled much of the continent.

No one is certain just when the first Old World disease organisms made the leap from Europeans to native Americans, but it seems likely that it occurred well before the first documented outbreak of smallpox on Hispaniola in 1518. Indirect evidence suggests that some serious illness may have arrived with the 1500 colonists who accompanied Columbus's second expedition in 1493. Of the seven Amerindians returning to Hispaniola after having been taken to Spain, five died en route home. In addition, Columbus reported that during the voyage, many Europeans, himself included, had fallen ill with an undisclosed malady. And by the end of 1494, disease and famine had claimed two-thirds of the Spanish settlers. Of the 550 Amerindian slaves seized by Columbus and shipped back to Spain in 1494, 200 died during the voyage and many of the survivors were sick upon debarkation.[1] Scholars have posited diagnoses of swine flu or typhus as the agents responsible for Spanish mortality, but whatever the disease, it could easily have spread to the native population of the island.[2] Las Casas included illness, along with starvation and warfare, among the disasters responsible for the precipitous decline of Hispaniola's native population between 1494 and 1496. And he claimed that "there did not remain of the multitudes of peoples that were on this island from the year of 1494 until that of 1496, it is believed, the third of all of them."[3] Accounts of Columbus's subsequent expeditions in 1498 and 1502 also include frequent mention of famine and disease among both Spaniards and natives.[4] Thus Hispaniola's large indigenous population had already experienced significant reduction even before the first smallpox epidemic began in 1518.

During the first decade of the sixteenth century, more than two hundred ships crossed the Atlantic; on board were thousands of European settlers and their microorganisms. By 1510, some ten thousand Europeans resided on the island of Hispaniola, significantly increasing the opportunities for the transfer of infection. During this same period, epidemic disease was rampant in southern Spain, the origin of most settlers, where an estimated one hundred thousand died of plague in 1507. Physicians reported outbreaks of an illness they labeled *modorra* throughout Spain between 1502 and 1507.[5] With so much disease circulating among Iberian populations, it is almost certain that one or more of these infections accompanied the growing numbers of colonists on their transatlantic crossings. In

1514, an illness identified as modorra broke out shortly after the expedition of Pedro Arias de Avila reached Central America; more than half of the fifteen hundred settlers died from illness and famine within a short time.[6] Because descriptions of modorra are vague, diagnosis remains difficult, but one scholar has argued that typhus or severe influenza accompanied by pneumonia appears to be the likely cause of this epidemic. Either disease could have easily spread to native populations.[7]

The Smallpox Epidemic of 1518

In 1520, the Dominican priest Bartolomé de las Casas described the devastation wrought by the first outbreak of smallpox in the Americas:

> A terrible plague came, and almost everyone died, very few remained alive. This was smallpox, which was given to the miserable Indians by some person from Castille; the feverish Indians, who were accustomed, when they could, to bathing in the rivers, threw themselves in anguish into the water, sealing the illness into their bodies, and so, as it is a destructive disease, they die in a short time: adding to this are the weakness and hunger and the nudity and sleeping on the floor and overwork and the little health care that those they serve have always taken. Finally, the Spanish seeing that the Indians were dying, began to feel the shortage [of labor], for which they moved to take some action to aid them, although it proved too little, because they should have begun it many years earlier; I do not believe that 1000 souls escaped this misery, from the immensity of people that lived on this island and which we have seen with our own eyes.[8]

The fact that smallpox had not arrived in the New World sooner is not surprising since the virus requires only three weeks to complete its cycle—a ten- to twelve-day incubation period, followed by the onset of illness, including the appearance of a deep-seated rash, lasting about two weeks. Thus lengthy transatlantic voyages, and the immunities that most Europeans had acquired to the illness as a result of childhood infections, delayed the arrival of smallpox in the Americas for a quarter of a century. According to one contemporary source, the Spanish historian Oviedo, this first epidemic of smallpox coincided with the forced resettlement of natives into communities close to Spanish towns.[9] In response to population decline and labor shortages, Spanish officials implemented a policy of resettlement in order to facilitate their access to those natives who remained scattered across the island. But congregating Amerindians into Spanish-controlled settlements increased the density of population and placed the natives in closer proximity to Europeans and their diseases, ultimately raising mortality rates and hastening the spread of illness across the island.

Once these diseases were unleashed upon the native population of Hispaniola, mortality rates soared: immediately following the epidemic, several observers testified that between one-third and one-half of the population had perished.[10] One witness, Hernando Gorjon, attributed the population crisis to "the great epidemic of smallpox and measles and respiratory ailments and other illnesses that the Indians of this island have experienced."[11] Since other diseases, particularly respiratory infections such as pneumonia, frequently accompany or follow outbreaks of smallpox, Gorjon's description is probably accurate. In many instances, these secondary infections proved as lethal as the smallpox virus, claiming the lives of those who might have recovered from the primary illness.

According to Las Casas and Oviedo, from Hispaniola the epidemic spread to Puerto Rico, Jamaica, and Cuba, leaving so few alive "that it seemed a great judgment from heaven."[12] In fact, by the middle of the sixteenth century, mistreatment and disease had reduced the native peoples of the Caribbean by more than 90 percent.

From the islands, the disease may have traveled to the Yucatán Peninsula, where contemporary sources noted an outbreak of smallpox during the second decade of the century.[13] But we know for certain that smallpox appeared on the Mexican mainland in April or May of 1520. The virus arrived with the expedition of Panfilo de Narvaez, dispatched by the governor of Cuba to arrest Hernán Cortés, the soon-to-be conqueror of the Mexica. While some claim that an African slave carried smallpox to mainland Mexico, an eyewitness, the Spanish official Vázquez de Ayllón, wrote that Cuban natives who accompanied the Narvaez expedition introduced the disease to the indigenous population of coastal Vera Cruz. While Vázquez de Ayllón did not remain in Mexico long enough to see the disease spread to the interior, he noted that smallpox "had caused great harm" in coastal areas.[14] Some years after the epidemic, Sahagún recorded the testimony of a native witness:

And [even] before the Spaniards had risen against us, a pestilence first came to be prevalent: the smallpox. It was [the month] of Tepeilhuitl when it began, and it spread over the people as great destruction. Some it quite covered [with pustules] on all parts— their faces, their heads, their breasts, etc. There was great havoc. Very many died of it. They could not walk; they only lay in their resting places and beds. They could not move; they could not stir;

they could not change position, nor lie on one side; nor face down, nor on their backs. And if they stirred, much did they cry out. Great was its destruction. Covered, mantled with pustules, very many people died of them. And very many starved; there was death from hunger, [for] none could take care of [the sick]; nothing could be done for them.[15]

Following the Spaniards' retreat from Tenochtitlán on June 30, 1520, the disease appeared in the capital; by the time the Spanish regrouped and returned to besiege the city, many thousands of natives had died, including the newly elected emperor, Cuitlahua, and other political and military leaders. Several months after his troops had captured the Mexica capital, Cortés described the deaths of many chiefs, explaining that they were caused by "the smallpox distemper which also enveloped those of these lands like those of the islands." Cortés's comparison of Mexican mortality to that of the Caribbean reveals, if only implicitly, the severity of population loss.[16] The power vacuum that resulted from the decimation of the Mexica leadership led to a breakdown of imperial authority, and as a result, many former tributaries chose to ally themselves with the Spanish. During the seventy-five days during which Cortés and his troops laid siege to Tenochtitlán, warfare and famine, as well as smallpox and other diseases, claimed thousands more lives. Cortés chose to

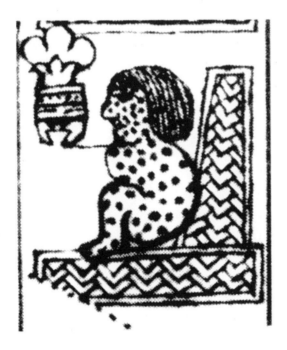

Fig. 10.
The earliest-known drawing of a Mexican smallpox victim by a native artist, about 1557. (Codex en Cruz, Bibliothèque Nationale, Paris)

claim the glory of Spanish victory over the Mexica for himself, but in his struggle a viral ally had served him at least as well as his military skills.[17]

Memories of Mexico's first smallpox epidemic remained strong long after the outbreak had ended; one scholar compiled twenty-six sources, some contemporary, others written many years after 1520, that refer directly to the epidemic and its impact.[18] This large number of references, made over the course of many generations, indicates the severity of mortality and the horror with which both Europeans and natives regarded this particular incident. During the next three centuries, major epidemics occurred frequently, but few remained in the public consciousness to the degree that the epidemic of 1519–1520 did. And while many descriptions of the Mexicas' initial encounter with smallpox contain no references to the number of people who died, the conqueror Bernardino Vázquez de Tapia, who witnessed the devastation of the epidemic, claimed that "more than one-fourth died." Likewise, the Franciscan Toribio de Benavente o Motolinia stated that in many regions mortality ranged from one-third to one-half or more.[19]

From central Mexico, the virus may have spread south into Central America, where an epidemic claimed the lives of many Guatemalan natives in 1520–1521. Influenza, measles, and a combination of smallpox and pneumonic plague have all been suggested as possibilities.[20] But while diagnosis remains uncertain, the description recorded by the native authors of the *Annals of the Cakchiquels* leaves no doubt as to its destructiveness:

It happened that during the twenty-fifth year [1520] the plague began, oh, my sons! First they became ill of a cough, they suffered from nosebleeds and illness of the bladder. It was truly terrible, the number of dead there were in that period. The prince *Vakaki Ahmak* died then. Little by little heavy shadows and black night enveloped our fathers and grandfathers and us also, oh, my sons! when the plague raged. It was in truth terrible, the number of dead among the people. The people could not in any way control the sickness. . . . Great was the stench of the dead. After our fathers and grandfathers succumbed, half of the people fled to the fields. The dogs and vultures devoured the bodies. The mortality was terrible. Your grandfathers died, and with them died the son of the king and his brothers and kinsmen. So it was that we became orphans, oh, my sons! So we became when we were young. All of us were thus. We were born to die![21]

Whether or not smallpox continued south into Honduras, Nicaragua, and Panama is not clear, but an official document written in Panama in 1527 referred to the "smallpox [that] had killed off the Indians there."[22] The northern trajectory of the epidemic is even more difficult to ascertain. Archaeological and historical records indicate that extensions of the smallpox epidemic of 1519 reached as far north and west as the Tarascan empire in Michoacán, but there is no evidence that it spread to native populations farther north.[23]

Some scholars have argued that in the decade following its introduction to the Caribbean, smallpox became pandemic, spreading throughout large sections of the Americas, even reaching as far south as the Andes.[24] While some evidence supports this thesis, vague and conflicting testimony from witnesses renders it far from certain. Both Spanish and Inca chroniclers recorded the impact of an epidemic that occurred several years before the arrival of Europeans. According to the Inca author Garcilaso de la Vega, the Inca ruler Huayna Capac died in Quito in 1524 after contracting a *chucchu* (chill) and *rupa* (fever).[25] The Spanish conqueror Miguel Cabello Balboa also attributed the death of Huayna Capac to a fever that coincided with a deadly epidemic in the Cuzco region. Sarmiento de Gamboa agreed that "an illness of fevers" was responsible but added that "others say it was smallpox and measles."[26] But Cieza de León, who traveled widely throughout the Andes during the 1530s and 1540s, claimed that in 1527 Huayna Capac was in the Quito area when he heard about Spanish ships off the coast. Shortly thereafter the Inca died in "a great epidemic of smallpox" that swept through the Andes.[27] The Jesuit Bernabé Cobo also claimed that an epidemic of smallpox broke out soon after Europeans began exploring the Peruvian coast.[28] Native chronicler Juan Santa Cruz Pachacuti described the epidemic as "measles," while Guaman Poma de Ayala identified it as "measles and smallpox."[29] The appearance of spots on the faces and bodies of victims lends support to the diagnosis of one of these infections.[30]

Given the timing of the outbreak, sometime between 1524 and 1527, several years after the introduction of smallpox into central Mexico and Guatemala and perhaps a year or two after its arrival in Panama, it appears more likely that this disease was responsible for the Andean epidemic. Furthermore, the first recorded outbreak of measles in the Americas did not occur until 1531.[31] From Panama the smallpox virus could have continued south in advance of Europeans, across the isthmus and into the Andes. Yet another possible route of transmission was provided by the ever-increasing number of Europeans on the Pacific coast of South America from 1524 on. One scholar has argued that the epidemic may have originated in Ferdinand Magellan's stopover in the Rio de la Plata area, then spread east along native trade

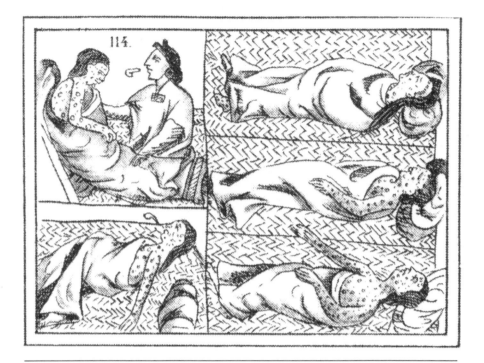

Fig. 11. *Mexican natives ill with smallpox. (Florentine Codex, 1590)*

routes.[32] Years later native informants emphasized the destructiveness of this epidemic in their testimony to Spanish officials. Cieza de León provided the only estimate of mortality, claiming that "more than 200,000 persons died," but it seems likely that if in fact smallpox was the disease responsible for the outbreak, the number of deaths was considerably greater.[33]

Mexico

The arrival of smallpox in 1520 was only the first in a series of virgin soil epidemics that developed in Mexico during the sixteenth century. Close on the heels of smallpox came other deadly pathogens, including measles, bubonic plague, and new strains of typhus and influenza. But the first outbreaks of these other infections were less clearly demarcated than that of smallpox, rendering diagnoses much less certain. In Mexico, contemporary sources noted widespread illness and death in both 1531 and 1532. Many scholars have argued that the 1531 incident may have marked the first outbreak of measles in central Mexico. One source claimed that mortality was especially high among children, but in a population that had never experienced the disease, one would expect many deaths among all age groups, not just the young. Thus it is far from certain that an epidemic of measles occurred in 1531.[34] Native chroniclers also reported an epidemic of *zahautl*, or smallpox, in 1532. But claims that many old people died undermine this diagnosis because the elderly, who survived the initial epidemic of smallpox in 1520, would have acquired immunity to the infection and therefore should not have been among the victims of this particular outbreak.[35] Once again, it is impossible to tell with any degree of certainty what disease was responsible for the epidemic of 1532. Perhaps the diagnoses should be reversed. Given the evidence, scant though it is, one might argue that many children died in 1531 as a result of contracting smallpox, while the outbreak a year later was caused by measles, which as a new disease would have affected all age groups, including the elderly.

Arguably the worst epidemic to strike central Mexico during the sixteenth century occurred between 1545 and 1548. While descriptions of mortality vary greatly, all agree that the number of deaths was

Table 3.1 Epidemics in Mexico, 1520–1595

Date	Disease	Mortality	Source
1520–1521	smallpox	"more than one-fourth died"; "one-third to one-half or more"	Vázquez, 148; Motolinia, 294
1531–1532	measles and/or smallpox	especially high among children and the elderly	Motolinia, 22; Prem, 30–31
1545–1548	matlazahuatl—typhus?	60–90 percent	Motolinia, 413; Prem, 31–34
1550	mumps	?	Prem, 34–35
1559–1560	influenza or diphtheria?	?	Prem, 35–38
1563–1564	measles	?	Prem, 37–38
1576–1581	typhus or bubonic plague?	"More than one-half died"	Paso y Troncoso, 12:86
1587–1588	cocoliztli	?	Prem, 42
1595	measles	?	Prem, 43

extraordinarily high. Symptoms of the matlazahuatl, as the Indians called it, included nosebleeds, fever, and bleeding from mucous membranes; the infection struck the native population regardless of age or class. The Spanish priest Motolinia claimed that 60 to 90 percent of the native population perished.[36] Scholars have most often diagnosed the disease as typhus, but once again, that is far from certain.[37]

In 1550, witnesses described an outbreak of disease the symptoms of which included swelling of the neck and high fever, probably mumps; they also claimed that many deaths ensued, probably from secondary complications.[38] Widespread sickness, possibly related to an outbreak of influenza or diphtheria, also appears in the record for 1559–1560 and again between 1563 and 1564. Measles may have been the disease responsible for the latter outbreak.[39]

Following the absence of major outbreaks of disease for more than a decade, one of the three worst epidemics of the sixteenth century began in April 1576, extending from Yucatán to northern Mexico. The illness or illnesses, which afflicted Africans and Europeans as well as natives, lingered until 1581. The most often noted symptom was hemorrhaging from body orifices, but sources also mentioned high fever and intestinal pain, followed by death in six or seven days. According to contemporary sources, mortality was very high, with one witness claiming that more than half of the remaining native population had perished.[40] Another source claimed that three hundred thousand to four hundred thousand had died by the end of the first year.[41] Once again, typhus is the most often cited diagnosis, but the symptoms could also indicate bubonic plague.[42] Repeated outbreaks of disease occurred throughout the remainder of the sixteenth century, but none as serious or as widespread as that of 1576–1581. And during the seventeenth century, regional epidemics were recorded for virtually every decade.[43]

Estimates of the degree of population decline in Mexico during the first century following the arrival of Europeans and their diseases range from an improbably low 25 percent to a high of over 90 percent. The wide discrepancy between these figures reflects disagreement over the size of the precontact population and regional rates of decline. Nevertheless, all agree that by the end of the sixteenth century, the native population had declined to somewhere between 1.1 and 3.5 million. In any case, the impact of Old World disease on the natives of Mexico was devastating. Based on a thorough review of the demographic literature and taking regional variations into account, it appears that Mexico's native population declined by 75 to 90 percent during their first century under Spanish colonial rule.[44]

Central America

The authors of the *Annals of the Cakchiquels* poignantly described the "heavy shadows and black night" that descended upon the Maya with the epidemic of 1520–1521. When Spanish troops, fresh from the conquest of Tenochtitlán, arrived in Guatemala under the command of Pedro de Alvarado, they encountered a native population already weakened and significantly diminished by disease. In the years that followed, Europeans and their diseases spread throughout Central America, further reducing the native population. In addition to numerous local outbreaks, historians have documented four more major epidemics in Guatemala before the end of the sixteenth century.[45] One of the worst occurred from 1532 to 1533, when measles, reported to have originated in Mexico, arrived in Guatemala. According to Alvarado, writing to the king of Spain in September 1532:

> All that remains for me to tell Your Magesty is that, throughout New Spain, there passed a sickness that they say is *saram pion,* one which struck the Indians and swept the land, leaving it totally empty. It arrived in this province some three months ago and, on my instructions, arrangements were made so that the Indians would be better cared for, so that they would not die in such great numbers as in all other parts. It was not possible to act before many died, so in all these parts also there has been a very great loss, for many indeed are dead."[46]

This was followed, in 1545, by a disease the Indians called *gucumatz,* apparently the same illness Mexicans named matlazahuatl.[47] And even though Spanish officials failed to confirm its presence in the region, other witnesses testified that mortality rates were very high: one Spaniard stated that three-fourths of the remaining native population perished.[48] While it is possible that this outbreak was an extension of the Mexican epidemic often diagnosed as typhus, others argue that it was pneumonic plague, an especially lethal form of the disease, spread by airborne droplets.[49] Mortality rates associated with pneumonic plague often reach 100 percent of those infected.

Between 1558 and 1562, epidemic disease, combined with famine, continued to decimate Guatemala's native population. Once again the native writers of the *Annals of the Cakchiquels* recorded the suffering and death:

> In the sixth month after the arrival [1560] of the Lord President [Juan Nunez de Valdecho] in Pagan, the plague which had lashed

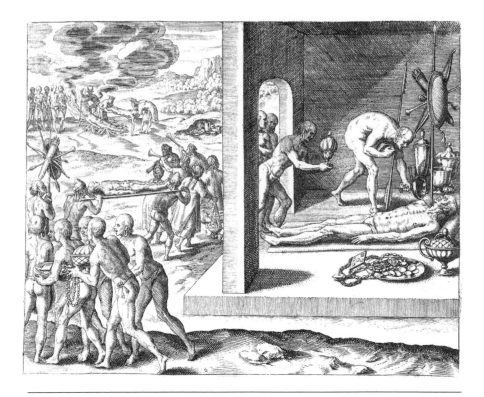

Fig. 12. *Mexican natives bury a dead nobleman. (Engraving by Theodore de Bry, 1590)*

the people long ago began here. Little by little it arrived here. In truth a fearful death fell on our heads by the will of our powerful God. Many families [succumbed] to the plague. Now the people were overcome by intense cold and fever, blood came out of their noses, then came a cough growing worse and worse, the neck was twisted, and small and large sores broke out on them. The disease attacked everyone here. . . . Seven days after Christmas the epidemic broke out. Truly it was impossible to count the number of men, women, and children who died this year. . . . Sickness and death were still rampant at the end of the sixty-third year after the revolution [May 18, 1562].[50]

While some have cited typhus and smallpox as the disease agents that caused the skin eruptions, most scholars agree that the symptoms best describe measles.[51] In addition, influenza may also have been a factor in this particular outbreak.[52] Yet another major epidemic occurred during 1576 and 1577, when smallpox, measles, typhus, and other illnesses arrived simultaneously from Mexico, and once again mortality rates were very high.[53]

South of Guatemala, in Honduras, Nicaragua, and Panama, Old World diseases also triggered significant population decline. And while information regarding the incidence of disease in this region is especially sparse,

Table 3.2 Epidemics in Central America, 1520–1578				
Location	Date	Disease	Mortality	Sources
Guatemala	1520–1521	smallpox	?	Lovell (1985), 60–68
Panama	1527	smallpox	?	Newson (1986), 128
Nicaragua	1529	smallpox?	?	Newson (1982), 278
Honduras and Nicaragua	1531	bubonic or pneumonic plague?	?	Newson (1982), 279; Newson (1986), 128; MacLeod (1973), 98
Guatemala	1532	measles	?	Lovell (1985), 68–71
Honduras and Nicaragua	1533	measles	?	Newson (1982), 280; Newson (1986), 129
Guatemala	1545	gucumatz— typhus or pneumonic plague?	"three-quarters died"	Lovell (1975), 71
Guatemala	1558–1562	measles and influenza	?	Lovell (1985), 72–75
Guatemala	1576–1577	smallpox, measles, and typhus	many children died	Lovell (1985), 75–78
Nicaragua	1578	?	?	Newson (1982), 280

documents record outbreaks in 1531, 1533, and 1578. Before 1530, the effects of disease appear by inference only: the previously mentioned reference to smallpox, which had reduced the native population of Panama by 1527, and a reference from 1529 to the depopulation of the mining centers of San Andres and Gracias a Dios due to illness.[54] Both plague and pneumonic plague have been suggested as possible pathogens responsible for the epidemic that developed in Honduras and Nicaragua in 1531. Symptoms included fever as well as pains in the side and stomach.[55] The illness, whatever it was, moved south, prompting the governor of Panama to write in May of that year:

> From a ship that has arrived from Nicaragua the *pestilencia* has struck this land, and it has been so great that although it has not yet ended, two parts of all the people that there are in this land have died, native Indians as well as slaves, and among them some Christians. I attest to Your Majesty that it is the most frightening thing that I have ever seen, because even the strongest does not last more than a day and a half, and some two or three hours, and now it reigns as at the beginning, and has become concentrated in Panama. The clerics are organizing processions, and praying, but not even these pleas to Our Lord have lifted his ire, to the point that I don't think there will remain alive a single person in all the land.[56]

Two years later, in 1533, a major outbreak of measles occurred in Honduras and Nicaragua. According to the seventeenth-century Spanish historian Antonio Herrera:

> At this time there was such a great epidemic of measles in the province of Honduras spreading from house to house and village to village, that many people died; and although the disease also affected the Spaniards . . . none of them died. . . . This same disease of measles and dysentery passed to Nicaragua where also many Indians died.[57] Observers claimed that one-third of Nicaragua's natives perished in this incident, while one-half of those in Honduras succumbed.[58]

The only other direct reference to outbreaks of disease during the sixteenth century comes from Nicaragua in 1578. This incident, which reportedly affected both Spaniards and Indians with a cough, may have been an extension of the epidemic that struck Guatemala the year before.[59] The precipitous decline of native populations throughout Central America during the sixteenth century indicates that disease continued to exact a heavy toll. But one scholar has argued that typhus and plague, frequently mentioned as the pathogens responsible for soaring mortality rates in highland areas of Mexico and Guatemala, were unsuited to the tropical conditions of Honduras, Nicaragua, and Panama; therefore these diseases may have played little or no role in the depopulation of this region.[60]

Estimates of the degree of demographic decline among the native peoples of Central America during the sixteenth and seventeenth centuries range from 80 to 90 percent in Guatemala to 92 percent in Nicaragua, except for the Nicoya Peninsula, where the number of Indians dropped some 80 percent owing to a greater degree of isolation and less penetration by the Spanish.[61] In Honduras, up to 95 percent of the native population had perished by 1550. The combined effects of a large Indian slave trade and epidemic disease accounted for the excessively high rates of depopulation in both Honduras and Nicaragua.[62]

The Andes

The possibility exists that in addition to the first epidemic of smallpox that probably struck between 1524 and 1527, at least one other epidemic may have swept through the Inca empire before the Spanish conquest, although no description remains. The previously mentioned epidemics of bubonic plague and measles that appeared in Central America in 1531 and 1533 could have arrived in the Andean area either overland from Panama or with an infected European seaman. Between 1531 and 1533, several expeditions arrived on the coasts of Peru and Ecuador, providing ample opportunity for the introduction of infection.

The first major Andean epidemic witnessed by Spaniards began in 1546. According to Cieza de León:

> A general pestilence spread throughout all of [the viceroyalty of] Peru, beginning south of Cuzco and covering all of the land; countless people died. The illness began with a headache and high fever, and later the headache passed to the left ear, and the disease was so severe that most of the sick died within two or three days.[63]

Some have diagnosed this outbreak as typhus, arguing that it could have been an extension of the matlazahuatl epidemic that had swept through Mexico a year earlier.[64] That no mention is made of the rash associated with typhus is not unusual because the eruption normally appears on the fifth or sixth day, and in this instance, many victims did not survive that

Table 3.3 Epidemics in the Andes, 1524–1591			
Date	Disease	Mortality	Source
1524–1527	smallpox	one-third to one-half died; "more than 200,000 persons died"	Cieza (1984), 1:219; Dobyns (1963), 494–97; Cook (1981), 70
1531–1533	measles or bubonic plague?	25–30 percent	Dobyns (1963), 497–99; Cook (1981), 70
1546	pneumonic plague or typhus	"innumerable people died," possibly 20 percent	Cieza (1984), 1:36; Dobyns (1963), 499–500; Cook (1981), 70; Newson (1995), 10–12
1558–1559	smallpox, measles, and influenza	15–20 percent	Espada, 2:205; Dobyns (1963), 500; Cook (1981), 70
1585–1591	smallpox, measles, typhus, and influenza	approximately one-half	Levillier, 11:207, 221, 284–85; Dobyns (1963), 501–8; Cook (1981), 70

long. There are, however, additional reasons for suspecting that a disease other than typhus was responsible: high fever, headache, and sudden death are all characteristics of pneumonic plague. A simultaneous epizootic among Peru's sheep and llama populations lends further credence to the diagnosis of plague because these animals are also susceptible to the plague bacillus.[65]

Twelve years later, in 1558, "a general epidemic of smallpox killed many Indians" in the Quito area.[66] In Peru, witnesses attributed the outbreak to smallpox and measles. This epidemic was made worse by the simultaneous appearance of a "severe cough," probably influenza, which claimed the lives of both Spaniards and Indians. This particular outbreak may have been an extension of the influenza pandemic that began in Europe in 1556. The virus reached Madrid in 1557; from there it could easily have been transported to the New World, where it raged in many regions, including Florida, Mexico, and Guatemala.[67] Recent studies of influenza epidemics indicate that children, the elderly, pregnant women, and individuals suffering from other infections such as smallpox are especially likely to develop severe cases of the disease, which may eventually lead to viral pneumonia and death.[68] It is estimated that in the Andes, between 15 and 20 percent of the native population died during this combined outbreak of smallpox and influenza.[69]

In spite of localized outbreaks of disease such as the unidentified illness that struck the mining center of Potosí, Bolivia, between 1560 and 1561, for almost thirty years, Andean residents enjoyed a respite from major epidemics.[70] Even though numerous illnesses remained endemic, the number of cases never warranted mention in either municipal or *audiencia* records. Thus a generation of natives grew up without exposure to many virulent strains of disease, and it was this generation that was most severely affected by the next wave of infection.

In April 1585, an epidemic of "measles and smallpox" began in Cuzco, spreading rapidly west to Huamanga and north to Lima. Amerindians proved especially susceptible to these two diseases, but a respiratory infection, probably influenza, followed in its wake, killing blacks and whites as well as natives. Approximately one-fifth of Lima's population perished during this initial wave of illness.[71] By February 1587, the outbreak had reached Quito and possibly beyond. Several months later, in July, another epidemic, moving in the opposite direction, struck the city. This second epidemic first appeared on the coast of Colombia in Cartagena and probably arrived with the expedition of Sir Francis Drake, which captured and occupied the city from January through February of 1586.[72] Drake's forces reportedly carried with them an infection contracted during a stopover at the Cape Verde Islands in November 1585. The disease, which appeared after they had been at sea for seven or eight days, produced a rash and fever and during the next three months claimed one-quarter of the ships' crews.[73]

Because these two epidemics overlapped in many areas, including Quito, some have assumed that the second was a continuation of the smallpox and measles episode.[74] But one scholar has argued that typhus appears more likely, given the prolonged period of mortality, suggestive of an insect vector. Also, epidemic louse-borne typhus has an incubation period of one to two weeks. Drake's expedition spent ten days on the Cape Verde island of Santiago, and the disease broke out after the men had been at sea for seven or eight days. Thus the timing of the epidemic is consistent with the diagnosis of typhus.

During the spring of 1589, epidemic disease returned with renewed virulence. Writing to the king of Spain in April, the viceroy described an epidemic of "smallpox and measles" that began in Quito and was spreading south into Peru. Once again, the initial wave of infection was followed by "a pestilential typhus," and the viceroy urged Spanish officials to use community funds to purchase food and medicine for the Indians. In that letter he also reported that "at the same time in the provinces of

Upper Peru [Bolivia] another illness of coughing with fever has struck and even though on some days in Potosí more than 10,000 Indians and some Spaniards are sick, until now no notable damage has resulted there or in Cuzco or Huancavelica."[75]

One month later, both epidemics converged on Lima, and though almost everyone became ill, few died.[76] That both Europeans and Creoles, American-born Spaniards, were also affected suggests that the disease that originated in Upper Peru was influenza. During June 1589, mortality rates rose again and the viceroy expressed alarm that in addition to natives and blacks, mulattoes, Creoles, and Europeans of all ages were also dying. The epidemic was especially severe north of Lima in the Trujillo Valley, and it seems likely that this outbreak of influenza continued its northern trajectory into the Quito area during the summer months.[77]

In the highlands of the audiencia of Quito this disease lingered, and in 1590 officials still reported many cases.[78] When the epidemics finally subsided the following year, they left behind a trail of death and destruction unsurpassed by even the 1546 episode. In 1591 caciques from the eastern lowland provinces of Yaguarsongo and Jaen testified that after the outbreak of smallpox, only a thousand natives remained of a population that had previously numbered thirty thousand.[79] Although the rate of demographic decline was not so severe in the highlands, approximately 50 percent of the native population perished.

The epidemics of 1585–1591 were only the last in a series of devastating encounters of native society with disease during the sixteenth century. Beginning with the arrival of smallpox in the 1520s, disease decimated Andean communities at irregular intervals from five to roughly twenty-five years. In each case, however, sufficient time elapsed after each episode to allow partial recovery of native communities. Then the next wave of disease struck, with individuals born since the last epidemic proving especially susceptible.

Review of the existing evidence, albeit incomplete, indicates that depending on the region, Andean populations reached their nadir somewhere between 1600 and 1650. By that time, the number of natives in the Andes had been reduced by approximately 75 to 80 percent.[80]

Many of the same epidemics that decimated highland populations in Colombia, Ecuador, and Peru also struck lowland communities along the coast. Colonial documents indicate that mortality rates were even higher here because of the frequent arrival of ships bearing newcomers. The infectious organisms that accompanied the new arrivals exposed these native populations to a greater variety of ills. The coastal population around the port of Guayaquil, for example, virtually disappeared by the end of the sixteenth century.[81] Although more isolated from Europeans and their diseases than coastal dwellers, natives of the eastern lowlands that extended into the Amazon Basin also suffered higher rates of mortality than highlanders. In both instances, native residents of these tropical areas, coastal and eastern lowlands, experienced higher rates of mortality in part because of complications stemming from an increased incidence of intestinal parasites and the insect-borne illnesses more common in warm climates.

Because of the problems inherent in colonizing the eastern lowlands— long distances from administrative and production centers, difficult terrain, and effective resistance from hostile natives—Spanish incursions were often transitory, leaving the region relatively isolated. It is impossible, therefore, to ascertain precisely when Old World infections first arrived there. The first references to large-scale depopulation due to epidemic disease date from the 1580s, but it seems likely that at least in some areas, Old World infections may have arrived earlier.[82] By the seventeenth century, however, Jesuit and Dominican missionaries were actively engaged in the colonization of the region, and their reports often noted the occurrence of epidemics and their demographic impact. For example, in the province of Mainas, situated in the eastern lowlands of Ecuador, epidemics of smallpox and measles occurred during the 1620s, 1640s, 1650s, 1660s, and 1680s, claiming more than half of the native population.[83]

To the north, in the highlands of Colombia, sixteenth-century documents record several epidemics beginning in the 1530s. Outbreaks that occurred in 1546, 1558, and 1585 coincided with epidemics in Ecuador and Peru and therefore may represent Andean pandemics.[84] Here, too, it is also possible that European diseases arrived even earlier. Cieza de León, who traveled through the Pasto area south of Bogota during the 1540s, wrote: "In the past the area must have been much more populated. . . . One cannot travel anywhere (except for the most broken and difficult [terrain]) without seeing that the land had been [previously] populated and worked."[85]

Demographic records for Colombia are sketchy, but those that do exist suggest that the native population declined by 75 to 90 percent, with significant regional variations.[86]

The Old World and the New

Similarities between the impact of virgin soil epidemics in the New World and the Old are significant and lend support to the argument that the experience of native American societies with imported epidemic diseases resembled that of human populations throughout Europe, Africa, and Asia. An examination of factors including cause, effect, and circumstance all reveal analogous situations on both sides of the Atlantic. First, as had so often been the case in the Old World, the arrival of virgin soil epidemics was precipitated by economically driven migration. During the second century, Roman imperialism facilitated the dissemination of smallpox throughout the Middle East and Europe, just as the political and economic expansion of the Mongols introduced bubonic plague to Europe and the Middle East in the fourteenth century. A century later, Europeans, searching first for a western sea route to Asia and later for access to the enormous human and natural resources of the New World, began arriving in ever-growing numbers on American shores. During the first century following contact, Europeans focused most of their efforts at colonization in the densely populated regions of the Caribbean and on the American mainland extending south from central Mexico. Thus it was in this vast region that Amerindian populations first experienced the onslaught of imported infections. And while the documentation regarding the disease history of the early sixteenth century is especially sketchy, evidence suggests that several outbreaks of imported infections, possibly a new strain of typhus or influenza, may have occurred before the first epidemic of smallpox erupted on the island of Hispaniola in 1518.

It is not clear whether the smallpox epidemic that began in the Caribbean in 1518 gradually spread to become pandemic or whether the disease was introduced into many regions by carriers wholly unassociated with the 1518 outbreak. In any event, virgin soil epidemics of smallpox could easily have propelled mortality rates as high as the 25 to 50 percent noted by contemporary observers Vázquez de Tapia and Motolinia. Thus a second similarity between virgin soil epidemics in the Old and New Worlds lies in the fact that mortality rates of 25 to 50 percent correspond closely with those recorded for similar outbreaks of smallpox in Athens in the fourth century BCE, in the Roman Empire during the second century CE, and in Japan during the eighth and ninth centuries. Even in modern times, when smallpox struck isolated populations during the nineteenth and twentieth centuries, mortality rates often reached 30 percent, and on the Indian subcontinent, where the disease has been endemic for many centuries, twentieth-century fatality rates often surpassed 20 percent among unvaccinated individuals.[87] In the New World after 1492, widespread violence, forced relocations, and the disruption of basic social service networks in many indigenous communities pushed mortality rates even higher.

A third similarity between the disease experiences of the Americas and the Old World was that the mortality associated with virgin soil epidemics was often greatly exacerbated by campaigns of military conquest. The epidemic of smallpox that first struck the Athenian army and then spread to the general populace in the fourth century BCE erupted during the turmoil and destruction of the Peloponnesian War, while Roman and Mongol military campaigns in the second and fourteenth centuries not only facilitated the spread of infectious diseases, but also exacerbated mortality rates as the result of widespread violence. Similarly, many of the epidemics that swept the Americas in the century following contact occurred during periods of intense military conflict between Amerindians and Europeans. Nicolas Federmann, a German visitor to Hispaniola in the 1520s, and Juan Sancho Paz Ponce de León, an administrator in the Ecuadorian province of Otavalo in the 1580s, emphasized that it was a combination of warfare, forced labor, and disease that led to the dramatic demographic decline of native populations in the Caribbean and the Andes. Throughout the Americas, wars of conquest led to higher mortality rates, not only as a result of large numbers of violent deaths, but also because of disruptions to food supplies, leading to widespread famines. In recounting the Spanish siege of Tenochtitlán in 1520, Cortés's secretary Francisco López de Gómara wrote, "And then came famine, not because of a want of bread, but of meal, for the women do nothing but grind maize between two stones and bake it. The women, then, fell sick of the smallpox, bread failed, and many died of hunger."[88] In fact, Sahagún claimed that more Mexica died of starvation than smallpox.[89]

Another significant factor in the history of virgin soil epidemics in both the Old and New Worlds was the development of significant regional variations in morbidity and mortality rates. Once again, the evidence is too scant to permit a nuanced interpretation of these patterns, but accounts indicate that the number of people falling ill and dying varied from one community to another. For example, Motolinia's statement that "in many provinces and towns half or more of the people died, and in others less than half, or a third part," illustrates the fact that not all communities experienced the same degree of devastation.[90] Factors affecting morbidity and mortality rates included the timing and duration of outbreaks. Epidemics that arrived during the planting or harvesting seasons or in conjunction with natural disasters such as droughts or flooding that reduced food supplies caused greater numbers of deaths than in communities that did not face these added stresses. And regions where epidemics raged for long periods of time, months as opposed to weeks, experienced significantly higher death rates.

But in spite of these important similarities, one major difference exists between the history of virgin soil epidemics in the New and Old Worlds, and that difference is of great significance. For only in the Americas and the islands of the Pacific did human populations experience the almost simultaneous arrival of several new infectious organisms, most notably smallpox, measles, and bubonic plague. In the Old World, each of these infections had reduced local populations by 25 to 50 percent, and even higher in some instances. In each case, stricken populations required at least three to four generations to recover demographically. In many areas of the Americas, however, native communities experienced repeated outbreaks of at least two of the three imported illnesses, all within the space of twenty to thirty years. In the most densely populated and highly developed regions of Mesoamerica and the Andes, smallpox arrived in the early to mid-1520s, followed by measles in the early 1530s, and possibly pneumonic plague or an especially severe form of typhus in 1545–1548. The arrival of just one of these diseases had plunged many populations in the Old World into severe demographic and social crises, but the almost simultaneous arrival of two or even three such lethal infections in combination with military conflicts and famines easily explains the staggeringly high mortality rates of the sixteenth century.

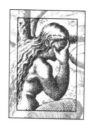

4 • Colonialism and Disease in Brazil and North America

As soon as I reached the aldeia [village] I found it all aflame with smallpox. I immediately ordered all the most dangerous cases gathered into one large hut, so that I could instruct and confess them. You cannot believe the trouble I had to confess one old woman who said she had not sinned.

João Felipe Betendorf,
*Chronica da missão dos Padres
da Companhia de Jesusno Estado do Maranhão*

News from the Gros Ventres, they say that they are encamped this side of Turtle Mountain, and that a great many of them have died of the smallpox—several chiefs among them. They swear vengeance against all the Whites, as they say the smallpox was brought here by the S.B. [steamboat].

F. A. Chardon,
Chardon's Journal at Fort Clark, 1834–1839

The Spanish were not alone in their attempts to profit from the tremendous wealth of the Americas: during the sixteenth century, numerous Portuguese, French, British, and Dutch expeditions also sailed to the New World. In 1500, Pedro Alvares Cabral explored the Atlantic coastline of Brazil, laying claim to that territory for the king of Portugal, and for the next several decades, Portuguese interest in the region focused on the export of a valuable dyewood that grew along the coast. Following several exploratory voyages along the coast of North America during the sixteenth century, the French gained control of the lucrative fur trade in the northeast and Great Lakes regions, and eventually New France encompassed a vast territory stretching from northern Canada to the Gulf of Mexico and from the Saint Lawrence River to west of the Mississippi.

Eager not to be left behind in the quest for American colonies, the early seventeenth century saw the arrival of Dutch settlers in the Hudson River Valley of New York and British settlers in Virginia. The British also colonized the Chesapeake Bay area and the region that became known as New England, beginning with the arrival of Puritan dissidents at Plymouth colony in 1620. Thus some 120 years after Columbus's arrival in the New World, the process of European colonization was well under way in many regions.

Unlike much of Mesoamerica and the Andean region of the Spanish empire, the areas colonized by the Portuguese, French, Dutch, and British differed in several respects. Most importantly for the purposes of this study, Brazil and North America were not home to highly developed civilizations such as those of the Mexica, Mayas, and Incas. As a result, the hunter-gatherer societies and chiefdoms of Brazil and North America boasted fewer inhabitants and lower populations densities. And while European contact with Brazil's coastal populations occurred at the beginning of the sixteenth century, in the rest of Brazil and throughout North America sustained contact developed later, during the seventeenth and eighteenth centuries. In addition, the colonial systems implemented by the Portuguese, French, Dutch, and British and their relations with conquered populations differed from those of the Spanish in significant ways that will be discussed in the next chapter. Thus levels of development, population densities, timing of contact, and colonial policies specific to each European nation determined the patterns of health and disease and the impact of epidemics in Brazil and North America.

Brazil

Because Portuguese colonization of Brazil was confined to coastal enclaves for much of the sixteenth century and because the number of immigrants to that region was smaller than the number of Europeans flocking to Spanish-controlled areas, fewer Europeans witnessed the arrival of Old World diseases, and therefore considerably less is known about their impact on the natives of Brazil. Nevertheless, by 1555, more than 350 ships carrying more than ten thousand Europeans had landed on the Brazilian coast, providing numerous opportunities for the introduction of Old World infections to that region's indigenous inhabitants, the Tupinamba.[1]

While no specific descriptions of virgin soil outbreaks in Brazil exist for the half century before 1550, the frequency of contacts between Europeans and Amerindians suggests that such incidents probably did occur. Making this development even more likely is the fact that European sailors often abandoned their sick comrades on shore to remove contagion from their midst, and when ill seamen were put ashore in populated areas, native residents would almost certainly have been exposed to whatever infectious organisms those individuals carried. And when infected sailors were not abandoned onshore, many crews routinely experienced outbreaks of a variety of diseases, including smallpox, influenza, dysentery, and typhus, thus increasing the likelihood of transmitting disease organisms to native populations. In at least one instance, records reveal that an infectious fever claimed the lives of many crewmen in the fleet of Sebastian Cabot as it sailed along the Brazilian coast in 1527.[2] While no evidence indicates that this particular outbreak spread to local

Table 4.1 Epidemics in Brazil, 1550–1600				
Location	Date	Disease	Mortality	Source
Bahia	1552	?	?	Hemming, 141
São Paulo	1554	fevers and hemorrhagic dysentery	?	Staden, 85–89; Hemming, 140
São Paulo to Bahia	1559–1561	fevers, hemorrhagic dysentery, and catarrh (possibly influenza)	at least 20 percent	Dean, 21; Hemming, 141–42
Bahia	1562–1563	smallpox and/or bubonic plague	30,000 natives died in first three months; one-quarter to one-third of survivors died subsequently	Dean, 22; Hemming, 142–43
Espirito Santo	1565	smallpox	?	Hemming, 144–45
Bahia	1575	smallpox and measles	?	Hemming, 175
Paraiba	1597	smallpox	10 to 12 deaths daily	Alden, 44–45

Tupinamba communities, the arrival of thousands of Europeans significantly increased opportunities for the transmission of Old World diseases to Brazil's coastal populations during the early years of European exploration. According to historian Warren Dean, the sparse population of the São Paulo coastline in the 1550s might be attributed, at least in part, to epidemics that went unreported.[3]

In addition, Portuguese colonial policies also facilitated the introduction of previously unknown infections to the region's inhabitants. Unlike Spain, Portugal permitted the legal enslavement of the native population, and especially after the founding of the first sugar plantations in the 1530s, the need for indigenous labor increased dramatically. The violence and dislocation occasioned by slave raiding most certainly provided many opportunities for the transmission of a variety of infectious organisms to Brazil's Tupinamba communities.

Permanent Portuguese settlement of the Brazilian coast began in the 1550s, and it is the observations of settlers and Jesuit missionaries that provide significant information on the impact of epidemics among the region's indigenous populations. While no details remain concerning the first recorded epidemic, an unidentified outbreak that erupted in 1552 near Bahia, considerably more information has survived on an epidemic of fevers and hemorrhagic dysentery that killed many Amerindians in the area of São Paulo in 1554. The published account of a German sailor, Hans Staden, held captive by the Tupinamba during this period, probably described this same epidemic. According to Staden, who was able to save his own life by convincing his captors that the god of the Christians had sent the epidemic to punish the Tupinambas for cannibalism, the disease claimed the lives of many Amerindians, but children and the elderly succumbed first.[4] Two years later, this same illness had reached the French colony at Rio de Janeiro, and according to one Frenchman, "This contagious malady ran everywhere so strangely that several of us died of it, and an infinite number of savages."[5] By 1559, fevers, respiratory infections (possibly influenza), and hemorrhagic dysentery had spread north to Espirito Santo, where some six hundred natives out of a population of three thousand died. From Espirito Santo, the epidemic continued its northern trajectory to Bahia, where it raged until 1561. The outbreak also reappeared in São Paulo that same year, claiming the lives of many thousands, especially children, who succumbed to the diseases within four or five days.[6] Throughout the epidemics of the 1550s, mortality rates were very high, especially among the many natives whose health had been seriously compromised by forced resettlement into Jesuit missions.[7]

In 1562, the first recorded epidemic of smallpox began, and while it is possible that the disease arrived earlier, to date, no evidence has been found to support this supposition. One scholar has suggested that this incident may have occurred simultaneously with an outbreak of plague, possibly introduced from Lisbon, where that disease had claimed forty thousand lives a year earlier.[8] According to the Jesuit Leonardo do Valle, writing from Bahia:

> When this tribulation [possibly referring to the epidemic of fever and hemorrhagic dysentery that ravaged the area in 1561] was past and they wanted to raise their heads a little, another illness engulfed them, far worse than the other. This was a form of smallpox or pox so loathsome and evil-smelling that none could stand the great stench that emerged from them. For this reason many died untended, consumed by the worms that grew in the wounds of the pox and were engendered in their bodies in such

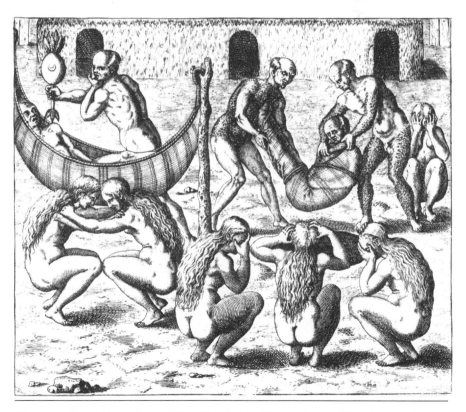

Fig. 13. *How the natives of Brazil fell sick. (Engraving by Theodore de Bry, 1592)*

abundance and of such great size that they caused horror and shock to any who saw them.[9]

Indigenous residents of the missions and those enslaved on Bahia's sugar plantations succumbed in large numbers, leading to severe labor shortages. As food supplies shrank, starvation threatened, further increasing mortality. According to Do Valle, "Driven by necessity, some went so far as to sell themselves for something to eat. One man surrendered his liberty for only one gourd of flour to save his life. Others hired themselves out to work all or part of their lives, others sold their own children."[10]

According to Jesuit reports, thirty thousand died during the first three months of the epidemic, and between one-fourth and two-thirds of the remaining population perished before the disaster subsided. Native converts also reported that smallpox had spread to Amerindian communities in the interior, claiming countless more lives.[11] By 1565, the epidemic had spread south to Espirito Santo, where one witness observed, "It was a pitiful spectacle. The houses served equally as hospitals for the sick and cemeteries for the dead. . . . You did not know which to pity most—to attend to the healing of the living, or to give the dead the common piety of a burial. The former called you with their cries, the latter with their pestiferous smell, piled four by four on top of each other, rotting and corrupt."[12]

In response to labor shortages, the Portuguese redoubled their efforts at slaving. Slave raids, in turn, facilitated the further spread of infections, and throughout the 1570s, disease and the violence associated with forced labor systems continued to reduce Brazil's indigenous population. In 1575, for example, an epidemic of smallpox and measles struck the missions of Bahia, killing many.[13] Smallpox also appeared along the northern coast again in 1597, claiming Europeans as well as natives.[14]

The rapidly declining supply of native labor prompted the Portuguese to begin importing large numbers of African slaves, and as a result, during the seventeenth and eighteenth centuries, between four thousand and fifteen thousand Africans per year entered Brazil. Along with this human cargo came numerous infections, most frequently smallpox, and studies indicate a close correlation between droughts, famines, and epidemics of smallpox in various parts of west Africa and subsequent outbreaks in Brazil. In some instances, sources directly attributed these outbreaks to recently imported Africans.[15] As a result of significant increases in both European and African immigration, during the first half of the seventeenth century, epidemics developed at least every two to five years. One of the worst outbreaks of the seventeenth century occurred in 1660, when smallpox erupted among the natives of Maranhao and Belem. According to the

Jesuit João Felipe Betendorf, "Maranhao was burning with a plague of smallpox. The missionary fathers often dug graves with their own hands to bury the dead, for there were aldeias [villages] where there were not two Indians left on foot. Parents abandoned their children and fled into the forests in order not to be struck by that pestilential evil." Betendorf also described his journey to the village of Cameta, where he went to hear the confessions of his sick parishioners:

> Three persons were missing who had fled into the forest. I sent repeatedly to summon them. They delayed, but our Good Lord permitted their enemies to shoot at them with arrows and wound some of their relatives, who then brought them to the aldeia. They were so covered in pox and putridity that they caused horror to their own families. When they saw that a Father wanted to confess them they told me not to approach, for the rotten smell they were giving off was intolerable. I rather feared that I would not hear them well, but it was God's pleasure that I heard them better than the others; and the rotten smell seemed to me like the smell of white bread when it is removed from the oven. To confess them I was forced to put my mouth close to their ears, which were full of nauseating matter from the pox, with which they were entirely covered.[16]

This same witness stated that the epidemic claimed the "greater part" of the natives, and in his description, he noted a problem frequently mentioned by Europeans: the tendency of infected natives to run away, thus spreading the disease to other communities. Widespread epidemics of smallpox also ravaged Brazilian populations during the 1680s and again in the 1690s.[17]

Throughout the seventeenth and eighteenth centuries, epidemics frequently spread into interior regions of Brazil, striking Amerindians residing in Jesuit missions in the Amazon and those farther south in Paraguay. One Jesuit, Father Sepp, described an epidemic of hemorrhagic smallpox that began in 1695:

> The force of the disease manifests itself in small pustules, like those that attack children in Europe or those that we develop during a high fever. Here the pustules are a terrible plague that invades the entire body and scarcely leaves any member intact. . . . [The disease] begins by attacking the throat and then the stomach. It burns the intestines with acute pains, and then completely dries the body fluids and causes loss of appetite and weakness of the

stomach. Thence comes the continuous flux of blood. With the blood [the disease] finally produces a corruption and evacuation of the intestines themselves. Even the eyes and ears are not spared: some lose their sight, others their hearing. This merciless plague might just be tolerable if it satisfied its fury on the adults alone; but it strikes even unborn children, expelling them with cruel anticipation from the maternal womb, in which nature should give them the right to nine months shelter.[18]

Because so much of the demographic decline of Brazil's native population occurred in remote regions beyond the purview of Portuguese colonialism, it is difficult to arrive at an estimate of the overall rate of depopulation. But owing to the colony's large traffic in Amerindian slaves and the descriptions of several epidemics, it is not unreasonable to assume declines of 75 to 90 percent during the first century after contact. Along the coast, however, demographic decline was even more severe; according to Dean, coastal Tupinamba populations "were nearly extinct" by 1600.[19]

North America

The native peoples of Greenland were the first to experience sustained contact with Europeans. During the five centuries between 1000 and 1500 AD, it is estimated that some seventy thousand Norse from Iceland and Norway lived in that region. Archaeological evidence clearly demonstrates that native Greenlanders and Europeans engaged in trade, and contemporary sources from Iceland and Greenland indicate that epidemics occurred in both areas during that five-hundred-year period. So while it appears likely that Paleo-Eskimo and Thule populations of Greenland and Labrador were the first to suffer from the introduction of Old World diseases, no direct evidence remains to support that conclusion.[20]

Plenty of evidence exists, however, to support the assertion that after 1492, the native societies of North America were repeatedly ravaged by epidemic infections, and throughout this vast area, French, English, and Dutch colonists frequently noted the devastating consequences of disease on indigenous communities. One of the earliest accounts to describe the impact of epidemic disease on the native population of North America was written by Thomas Hariot, who accompanied Sir Walter Raleigh's expedition to Roanoke Island in 1584:

Within a few dayes after our departure from everie such towne, the people began to die very fast, and many in short space; in some townes about twentie, in some fourtie, in some sixtie, and in one sixe score, which in trueth was very manie in respect of their numbers. . . . The disease was also so strange, that they neither knew what it was, nor how to cure it; the like by report of the oldest men in the countrey never happened before, time out of minde. A thing specially observed by us, as also by the naturall inhabitants themselves.[21]

Hariot's observations regarding the timing of outbreaks, significantly increased mortality rates, and the natives' unfamiliarity with the illness were repeated by many colonists who settled in regions all over North America during the next three centuries.

Florida and the Southeast

Spain's point of entry into North America was from the south. In 1513, Juan Ponce de León led a force from Hispaniola to explore the Atlantic and Gulf coasts of the land he called La Florida. Other Europeans followed, including those engaged in unofficial slaving expeditions. One of those, led by Pedro de Salazar sometime between 1514 and 1516, captured five hundred natives, two-thirds of whom died on the voyage to Hispaniola; the remainder reportedly died after landing.[22] While it is impossible to know what illness killed these natives, this incident coincided with the outbreak of modorra brought to Central America by the Pedro Arias expedition. In that instance, typhus or severe influenza was suspected, and they appear as likely possibilities in this case as well.

Other than the reference to the deaths of the natives captured by Salazar, no documentary evidence exists to elucidate the disease history of the southeastern United States during the sixteenth century. But that has not prevented scholars from arguing about whether or not epidemics of Old World origin arrived in the region before 1600. Based solely on inference and speculation, anthropologist Henry Dobyns argues that "eight serious epidemics in Colonial populations could rather easily have been transmitted from New Spain and/or Cuba to the Calusa and Timucua [of Florida]" between 1512 and 1562.[23] Dobyns includes among those extensions of the Mexican smallpox pandemic of 1520–1524, the matlazahuatl epidemic of 1545–1548, and the mumps epidemic of 1550. Relying on documentary and archaeological evidence, anthropologist Clark Larsen, on the other hand, mentions no outbreaks during the sixteenth century; rather, he cites unidentified epidemics in 1613–1617, 1649–1650, an outbreak of smallpox in 1655, and measles in 1659. He does concede, however, that more epidemics probably occurred.[24] The

Table 4.2 Epidemics in Florida, 1613–1659			
Date	Disease	Mortality	Source
sixteenth century	no direct evidence, but it is likely that epidemics did occur		Dobyns (1983), 275–90; Larsen (1992), 27; Milanich, 214–18
1613–1617	?	Europeans and natives died; 50-percent mortality in some native communities	Hann, 175
1649–1650	?	Europeans and natives died	Hann, 23
1655	smallpox	Africans and natives died	Hann, 176
1659	measles	10,000 natives died	Hann, 177

chronology of archaeologist Jerald Milanich agrees with that of Larsen, but he adds an unidentified epidemic in 1595.[25] While insufficient evidence exists to prove the occurrence of the epidemics cited by Dobyns, there is no doubt that certainly by the first decades of the seventeenth century, the number of Florida natives plummeted as a result of their numerous encounters with various European infections.

Records reveal that at least two outbreaks of disease occurred between 1613 and 1617, claiming the lives of both Europeans and Amerindians. According to a Spanish priest, "We find that from four years ago down to the present, there have died on account of the great plagues and contagious diseases that the Indians have suffered, half of them, in the which Your Magesty has had a very great part in the growth that was given to heaven."[26]

The unidentified epidemic of 1649–1650 also killed Europeans and natives alike, and the smallpox outbreak of 1655, which lasted ten months, infected Africans as well as the indigenous population. In 1659, the governor of Florida reported that some ten thousand natives had perished during a recent outbreak of measles.[27] Some evidence suggests that the remote location of the Apalachee of the western Gulf Coast area around Pensacola and the natives' hostile relations with Europeans may have protected them temporarily from the worst depredations of disease. But the creation of mission settlements during the seventeenth century ensured sustained contact and the eventual decline of the Apalachee.[28]

Dobyns has argued for a 95-percent decline in the number of natives in the first century following contact.[29] But another source put the decrease at 80 percent by 1675. This same author also claimed, however, that as a result of continued outbreaks of disease, mistreatment, and slavery, the Amerindian population of Florida had become extinct by the 1760s.[30]

In other regions of the southeast, disease also took a heavy toll. While evidence is scant for the period before 1700, when sustained contact developed between natives and Europeans, in the lower Mississippi Valley and in the interior of Georgia, Tennessee, and Alabama archaeologists have uncovered evidence of dramatic population decline during the sixteenth century.[31] In 1526 Lucas Vázquez de Ayllon led an expedition that attempted to establish a colony on the coast of South Carolina. Within six months, more than two-thirds of the five hundred settlers had died and the colony was abandoned. When members of the expedition of Hernando de Soto arrived there sometime between 1539 and 1543, they noted: "About this place, from half a league to a league off, were large vacant towns grown up in grass that appeared as if no people had lived in them for a long time. The Indians said that two years before, there had been a pest in the land, and that the inhabitants had moved away to other towns."[32] They also described "four large houses . . . filled with the bodies of people who had died of the pestilence."[33]

While it remains uncertain that the disease that caused this devastation was of Old World origin, such a pathogen could have been introduced into the region either by direct contact with Europeans or by diffusion from native populations in Florida or some other coastal area that had at least periodic contact with disease-carrying Europeans. Between the de Soto expedition and the end of the seventeenth century, the historical record regarding incidents of disease in the southeast remains blank until 1698, when a French missionary in Arkansas noted the effects of a smallpox epidemic that had recently passed through the region:

> It is not a month since they got over the small pox which carried off the greatest part of them. There is nothing to be seen in the village but graves. There were two (groups) together there and we estimated that there were not a hundred men; all the children and a great part of the women were dead.[34]

As contact between Europeans and Amerindians increased during the eighteenth century, travelers often commented on the sparseness of population throughout the region; this in marked contrast to the dense populations described by members of the de Soto force over a century before. In Louisiana, one observer noted the decline of local indigenous societies, adding that some had disappeared altogether.[35] In Virginia and the Carolinas, smallpox also began to make regular appearances toward the end of the seventeenth century, with particularly devastating outbreaks developing in 1667, 1679–1680, and 1696–1698.[36] According to historian Peter Wood, "The region's native population had already been suffering a steep decline for nearly two centuries [the sixteenth and seventeenth centuries], particularly among the coastal tribes. . . . Between 1685–1730, the South's native population was further reduced by a full two-thirds, from roughly 200,000 to fewer than 67,000. Warfare, enslavement, and migration, but most of all epidemic disease, ravaged the major peoples of the Southeast."[37]

The Southwestern United States and Northern Mexico

European contact with the native societies of the southwestern United States and northern Mexico began with the journey of Alvar Núñez Cabeza de Vaca, who along with three other survivors of an ill-fated expedition to Florida in 1529 crossed the continent from Tampa Bay into Texas and New Mexico, headed south through Sinoloa and Sonora, and eventually reached Mexico City in 1536. Three years later, in 1539, a Franciscan priest, Father Marcos de Niza, led an exploratory force into northwestern Sonora, southern Arizona, and the territory of the Zuni in present-day New Mexico. The expedition of Francisco Vázquez de Coronado followed in 1540. Sustained contact did not develop, however, until the founding of Jesuit missions during the 1590s.

Nevertheless, documentary evidence indicates that from the 1530s on, epidemics of Old World diseases regularly reached the native peoples of this remote region. Although northern populations probably escaped the ravages of the first smallpox epidemic that struck central Mexico between 1520 and 1524, a Spanish force led by Nuño de Guzman introduced dysentery, typhoid, and possibly malaria into Sinoloa and Sonora in 1530 with devastating results for Europeans and natives alike. In Nayarit and Sinoloa, an epidemic of measles raged from 1530 to 1534.[38] One source claimed that 130,000 Amerindians from Culiacán alone died as a result of contracting this infection, leaving only 20,000 survivors.[39] It also appears likely that much of the northern area escaped the terrible matlazahuatl epidemic that struck central Mexico from 1545 to 1548; documentary evidence indicates the disease did not extend beyond Zacatecas and Culiacán.[40]

The absence of references to incidents of disease between the 1540s and 1570s may indicate that northern populations enjoyed a respite from epidemic illnesses, but it is more likely that such events simply went

Table 4.3 Epidemics in the Southwestern United States and Northern Mexico, 1530–1700			
Date	Disease	Mortality	Source
1530s	dysentery, typhoid, measles, and possibly malaria	86 percent of the native population of Culiacán died	Tello, 250–51
1540s–1570s	no direct evidence, but occurrence of epidemics likely		
1576–1581	plague and/or typhus, typhoid and dysentery	?	Reff, 124–26
1587–1588	smallpox	?	Reff, 127
1593	smallpox and measles	in Sinoloa, two-thirds of children and one-half of adults died	Reff, 135
seventeenth century	number of epidemics increases following the arrival of Jesuits	?	Reff, 132–79

unrecorded owing to the small number of Spaniards in the region. But the northward expansion of the colonial silver-mining economy and the long-distance and local trade spawned by that sector eventually resulted in the regular introduction of many infectious agents. As a result, epidemics occurred with increasing regularity: plague and/or typhus, typhoid, and dysentery between 1576 and 1581; *cocoliztli*, possibly smallpox, in 1587 and 1588; and cocoliztli again in the 1590s.[41] Following the arrival of Jesuit missionaries in northwestern Mexico in 1591 and the subsequent creation of permanent mission settlements, the incidence of epidemics increased significantly, with outbreaks occurring frequently during the first half of the seventeenth century. In 1593, for example, an epidemic of smallpox struck the missions of Sinoloa, claiming the lives of two-thirds of infants and children and one-half of all adults.[42] Epidemics continued during the remainder of the colonial period, "but demographic data indicate most native populations largely were destroyed by 1678."[43]

Documentation regarding the occurrence of disease in areas farther north, among the Pueblo peoples of Arizona and New Mexico, for example, is even more scant. The first Spanish colony in this region was founded in 1598, and between 1600 and 1643, half of the Pueblo's settlements were abandoned.[44] The first recorded epidemic of smallpox occurred in 1636, but it is likely that Old World diseases reached the area several decades earlier: another outbreak of an unnamed infection erupted in 1640.[45] Reporting of epidemics improved during the eighteenth century, but the lack of data for the remainder of the seventeenth century should not be interpreted as the absence of major outbreaks of disease. The Pueblo Revolt in 1680 destroyed many documents that may have contained information regarding disease patterns in the area. It was not until the reconquest of the area in 1696 that regular record keeping was reestablished. Thereafter, mission documents include references to at least twelve epidemics during the eighteenth century and at least nine during the nineteenth century.[46]

The Northeastern United States and Canada

By the end of the fifteenth century, commercial fishing boats were arriving off the coast of New England and eastern Canada in ever-increasing numbers. During the sixteenth century, the number of explorers and fishermen who sailed for eastern North America numbered in the thousands. But regular, sustained contact between natives and Europeans in this region did not develop until the early seventeenth century. Thus evidence for the introduction of Old World infections to the native peoples of the northeastern United States and Canada is nonexistent for the fifteenth and sixteenth centuries. One reference to an outbreak of disease among the Saint Lawrence Iroquois in 1535 by French explorer Jacques Cartier may describe influenza or some other respiratory ailment, but there is no indication that Amerindians contracted the infection from Europeans.[47] In 1608, another French explorer, Samuel de Champlain, wrote that dysentery and scurvy had claimed the lives of several natives. Then in 1611, he recorded the deaths of many Algonquins from "a fever that had broken out among them."[48] Again, no evidence suggests that the diseases responsible for these casualties were of Old World origin. Nevertheless, because of the frequency of contact between natives and Europeans, it is possible that infectious organisms were introduced into indigenous populations early in the sixteenth century.

The first reference to the fact that introduced diseases had already taken their toll among native populations comes from a Jesuit account written in 1616, referring to an incident that took place among the Micmac of Nova Scotia between 1611 and 1613

[The natives] are astonished and often complain that, since the French mingle and carry on trade with them, they are dying fast and the population is thinning out. For they assert that, before

Table 4.4 Epidemics in the Northeastern United States and Canada, Seventeenth Century			
Date	Disease	Mortality	Source
1608	dysentery and scurvy	?	Carlson et al., 147
1611	fever	?	Carlson et al., 147
1611–1613	pleurisy and dysentery	?	Thwaites, 3:105
1616–1619	smallpox?	over 75 percent died	Adams, 1:9–11; Bratton, 351–83
1630s	smallpox	?	Bradford, 2:193–94; Cook, 493
1647	influenza?, dysentery, and tuberculosis	attacked both Europeans and natives	Cook (1973), 493–95
1640s on	localized epidemics of smallpox	?	Cook (1973), 493; Duffy, 43–69

this association and intercourse, all their countries were very populous and they tell how one by one the different coasts, according as they have begun to traffic with us, have been more reduced by disease.[49]

While the author of this passage failed to attribute population decline to particular disease agents, Jesuit documents elsewhere described "pleurisy, quincy (sore throat) and dysentery" among the Micmac.[50]

The first widespread epidemic of Old World origin to be witnessed by Europeans appeared in the region extending from central Maine to southern Massachusetts between 1616 and 1619. According to one observer writing in 1622:

[The natives] died on heapes, as they lay in their houses; and the living, that were able to shift for themselves, would runne away and let them dy, and let there Carkases ly above the ground without buriall. For in a place where many inhabited, there hath been but one left a live to tell what became of the rest; the livinge being (as it seems) not able to bury the dead, they were left for Crowes, Kites and vermin to pray upon. And the bones and skulls upon the severall places of their habitations made such a spectacle after my comming into these partes, that, as I travailed in the Forrest nere the Massachussetts, it seemed to mee a new found Golgotha.[51]

While many have written on the demographic impact of this deadly epidemic, the evidence does not permit a definite diagnosis of the disease responsible for this catastrophe. Sources describe headache, "spots" or lesions, and a yellow discoloration of the skin as characteristics of the illness. Mortality rates were very high, over 75 percent, suggesting that this was a virgin soil epidemic. Onset and progress of the disease were so rapid that many indigenous communities were unable to keep up with the soaring number of burials. In 1621, European colonists observed, "ther sculs and bones we found in many places lying still above the ground, where their houses and dwellings had been; a very sad spectacle to behold."[52] While the infection broke out several years before the arrival of Pilgrim colonists, other Europeans were already exploring the area and ample opportunities existed for the transmission of disease to the native population. Yellow fever, measles, typhoid, chicken pox, typhus, bubonic plague, cerebrospinal meningitis, and smallpox have all been mentioned as possible disease agents, and while we will never know for certain what the disease was, one author has made a convincing case for malignant confluent smallpox, a particularly virulent form of the disease in which the confluence of the pustules and the accumulation of pus under the skin produce a yellowish discoloration.[53] In any event, the epidemic claimed the vast majority of the region's native inhabitants, leading one observer to comment on the "ancient plantations, not long since populous, now utterly void." And according to one Plymouth chronicler, a local native informant had related "that about four years ago all the inhabitants died of an extraordinary plague, and there [was] neither man, woman, nor child remaining."[54] Thus when the Pilgrims arrived on the coast of Massachusetts in 1620, they encountered a native population greatly reduced by Old World disease. That the colonists and their descendents did not lament the decline of their new neighbors is illustrated by a statement written some eighty years later by the Reverend Cotton Mather, who noted, "The woods were almost cleared of those pernicious creatures, to make room for better growth."[55]

Other epidemics followed. In 1630 English passengers disembarking in Boston introduced smallpox to the area. Three years later the disease raged among the native population of Massachusetts, and by the following year it had spread into Connecticut and beyond. According to William Bradford, a leader of the Plymouth colony:

This spring, also, those Indeans that lived aboute their trading house there fell ill of the small poxe; and dyed most miserably; for a sorer disease cannot befall them; they fear it more then the plague; for usualy they that have this disease have them in abundance, and for wante of bedding and linning and other helps, they fall into a lamentable condition, as they lye on their hard mats, the poxe breaking and mattering, and runing one into another, their skin cleaving (by reason therof) to the matts they lye on; when they turn them, a whole side will flea of at once, (as it were,) and they will be all of a gore blood, most fearful to behold; and then being very sore, what with could and other distempers, they dye like rotten sheep.[56]

Smallpox also appeared among the Iroquois of the Hudson River Valley and the Hurons and Ottawa of the Great Lakes and Saint Lawrence River regions. In fact, between 1633 and 1641 smallpox was a constant presence among the native populations of New England and eastern Canada. According to Cook, "After the decade 1630–1640, small pox was never absent among the populations of eastern North America."[57]

In 1647, an epidemic of what may have been influenza attacked Amerindians and Europeans alike, spreading throughout New England. Observers also noted frequent outbreaks of dysentery and the increasingly destructive presence of tuberculosis among natives.[58] Other respiratory ailments such as pneumonia and influenza as well as measles, typhus, and syphilis also contributed to the decline of indigenous communities. But smallpox, characterized by many as endemic following the 1640s, appears to have posed the most serious threat to native health. This disease flared into localized epidemics in 1648–1649, 1658, 1664–1666, 1675, and 1689–1690 and continued to wreak havoc throughout the eighteenth century.[59] By all accounts, the epidemics of the seventeenth century devastated the Amerindian peoples of the Northeast, at least 75 percent of whom had perished by 1650; by the end of the century, only 5 percent of their precontact numbers remained.[60]

California and the Pacific Northwest

Only twelve years following the Spanish capture of Tenochtitlán, Europeans began exploring the territory that became known as Baja California. In fact, in 1535, Hernán Cortés himself arrived intent on conquest. In all, nineteen expeditions ventured into the area before permanent settlement began at the end of the seventeenth century. In 1542, Juan Rodríguez Cabrillo sailed up the coast of California as far as Santa Barbara, to be followed in succeeding years by other Europeans who pushed farther north. While sustained contact between natives and Europeans did not develop until the last years of the seventeenth century in Baja and even later in Alta, or Upper, California, Old World diseases could have been introduced either by explorers or by natives traveling trade routes that extended into central Mexico. But while ample opportunities for such transmission existed, no evidence suggests that such an event occurred. Nevertheless, the oral traditions of the Chumash of the Santa Barbara area record that shortly before the arrival of Europeans in the 1770s, an epidemic broke out among coastal inhabitants and "people went around feeling sick until they fell backwards, dead."[61]

Because of its great distance from the center of power in Mexico City, Spanish colonization of Baja California did not begin until 1697, when the first in a series of Jesuit missions was created at Nuestra Señora de Loreto; sixteen more missions followed by the middle of the eighteenth century. Spurred on by concerns about growing Russian and English expansion, Spain authorized the Franciscans to establish twenty-one missions along the coast of Alta California from San Diego to San Francisco between 1769 and 1823. Along with the missions came military units and civilian populations from New Spain. One of the major goals of the missions was to remove natives from their villages and relocate them within mission settlements. Vague evidence suggests the outbreak of epidemic disease shortly after the arrival of missionaries in the late 1760s: "The number of coastal Chumash baptized by the missionaries is about half the number Portola saw in 1769."[62] Parish registers maintained by the Franciscans clearly indicate that shortly after the creation of the missions, their native populations began to decline dramatically. Among mission populations, venereal diseases, tuberculosis, and dysentery posed a constant threat, and mortality rates were very high, especially among infants and children. The first recorded, but unidentified, epidemic occurred between 1790 and 1792, followed by outbreaks of typhoid and pneumonia in 1796 and diphtheria between 1800 and 1802. The first recorded epidemic of measles occurred in 1806, followed by another in 1821–1822 and a third in 1827–1828. Influenza claimed many lives in 1832, and epidemic smallpox was officially recorded for the first time in 1844.[63] Cook has argued for a decline of at least 80 percent in the post-contact period.[64] Among the once numerous Chumash of the Santa Barbara area, only two hundred survived by 1880.[65]

The introduction of Old World diseases also coincided with the arrival of European explorers in the Pacific Northwest. Here native accounts tell of the devastation caused by the arrival of smallpox in the late 1770s or early 1780s. According to one version:

One salmon season the fish were found to be covered with running sores and blotches, which rendered them unfit for food. But as the people depended very largely upon these salmon for their

Table 4.5 Epidemics in California, 1760–1884	
Date	Disease
1760s	unidentified outbreak
1790–1792	unidentified outbreak
1796	typhoid and pneumonia
1800–1802	diphtheria
1806	measles
1821–1822	measles
1827–1828	measles
1832	influenza
1844	smallpox

Sources: Walker, 419; Walker and Johnson (1992), 133–36; Walker and Johnson (1994), 110–14.

winter's food supply, they were obliged to catch and cure them as best they could, and to store them away for food. They put off eating them till no other food was available, and then began a terrible time of sickness and distress. A dreadful skin disease, loathsome to look upon, broke out upon all alike. None were spared. Men, women, and children sickened, took the disease and died in agony by hundreds, so that when the spring arrived and fresh food was procurable, there was scarcely a person left of all their number to get it. Camp after camp, village after village, was left desolate. The remains of which, said the old man, in answer to my queries on this head, are found today in the old camp sites or midden-heaps over which the forest has been growing for so many generations. Little by little the remnant left by the disease grew into a nation once more, and when the first white men sailed up the Squamish in their big boats, the tribe was strong and numerous again.[66]

Other oral traditions from the region also describe the widespread devastation that followed the arrival of the dreaded disease. Precisely where the epidemics originated and when they arrived is not clear, but the British explorer George Vancouver, who visited many coastal areas of the Pacific Northwest in the early 1790s, recorded seeing many abandoned settlements. Another member of the expedition recorded this observation of remains encountered in the Puget Sound:

> During this Expedition we saw a great many deserted Villages, some of them of very great extent and capable of holding many human Inhabitants—the Planks were taken away, but the Rafters stood perfect, the size of many a good deal surprised us, being much larger in girth than the Discovery's Main mast. A Human face was cut on most of them, and some were carved to resemble the head of a Bear or Wolf—The largest of the Villages I should imagine had not been inhabited for five or six years, as brambles and bushes were growing up a considerable height.[67]

While the cause of such widespread abandonment of villages was not clear to Vancouver and others, they did conclude that the region had been recently depopulated.[68] In addition, Vancouver and others noted that many natives displayed the scarring characteristic of smallpox. One wrote: "The smallpox most have had, and most terribly pitted they are; indeed many have lost their Eyes and no Doubt it has raged with uncommon Inveteracy among them but we never saw any Scars with wounds, a most convincing proof in my Mind of their peaceable Disposition."[69] Thus epidemics of Old World diseases had reached the Pacific Northwest sometime before the 1790s and in many instances preceded Europeans into the area.

Debate remains as to the origins of the disease, however. One theory holds that the outbreak of smallpox that devastated the Pacific Northwest during the 1780s began in central Mexico in 1782. Eventually the disease spread southward into Chile and north through New Mexico into the Great Plains and Pacific Northwest, where it caused great mortality among native populations.[70] Another possibility is that the disease originated in an epidemic that began in Alaska in 1769 and spread south down the coast.[71] Yet a third possibility also exists: that smallpox arrived among the crew of several Spanish ships that visited the region between 1774 and 1779.[72] In any case, once smallpox was introduced into native populations, the death tolls were staggering.

Smallpox returned to the region possibly as soon as 1801 but certainly in 1836–1838, 1853, and 1862–1863. Malaria was also introduced into the area sometime after 1830, triggering high mortality rates especially among children, who often died of complications.[73] In addition to devastation from smallpox and malaria, outbreaks of measles, influenza, and dysentery claimed many lives throughout the nineteenth century.

On the Columbia Plateau, epidemic disease also decimated the native population at the end of the eighteenth century. But recent archaeological findings suggest that infections of Old World origin may have entered the area as early as the first half of the sixteenth century.[74] The same epidemics of smallpox that devastated native communities along the Pacific coast during the 1770s probably struck inhabitants of the Columbia Plateau as well. It is also likely that a second, less virulent outbreak occurred in 1800–1801.[75] Thus by the time European fur traders arrived during the first decade of the nineteenth century, the indigenous population had already been reduced. Overall, estimates for the extent of the decline of native populations of the Pacific Northwest range from 80 to 90 percent.[76]

The Great Plains

While Coronado explored sections of the Great Plains in 1541, it was not until the first half of the eighteenth century that Europeans recorded renewed contact with the region's native peoples. First in 1723 and again in 1738, French fur-trading expeditions traveled among the Arikara and Mandan. But recent archaeological evidence indicates that Old World diseases probably arrived in the area early in the seventeenth century.[77] Excavations of Amerindian settlements situated in the Middle Missouri region on the border of North and South Dakota have yielded the remains of European trade goods, and coincident with their appearance is evidence of population decline, probably occasioned by the introduction of epidemic disease. In this case, disease could have reached Plains populations in two ways: Infection could have spread along native trade routes, most probably from the southwest, where epidemics occurred in 1638 and 1671, and/or disease organisms could have been introduced directly by European explorers and trappers who ventured into the region. A human skull, excavated from Swan Creek, South Dakota, has been identified as that of a Caucasian male, forty to fifty years old, probably French or Spanish. The remains date from the period 1675–1725, clearly indicating that whites were present in the area several decades before their presence was officially recorded. The archaeological record also indicates demographic recovery following the declines of the early seventeenth century.[78]

Sustained contact between Europeans and the indigenous inhabitants of the Plains, however, did not develop until the last quarter of the eighteenth century. Sometime around 1780, an epidemic of smallpox broke out among the populations of the Middle Missouri. Europeans who traveled through the region during the 1790s and early 1800s frequently noted the presence of abandoned villages. According to Jean Baptiste Truteau, a French trader who visited the Arikara during the spring of 1795

In ancient times the Ricara nation was very large; it counted 32 populous villages, now depopulated and almost entirely destroyed by the smallpox which broke out among them at three different times. A few families only, from each of the villages, escaped; these united and formed the two villages now here.[79]

In addition, epidemics of whooping cough and cholera reportedly occurred between 1832 and 1834.[80]

The first epidemic among natives of the northern Plains to be observed directly by whites began in July of 1837, when smallpox arrived with passengers on a steamboat cruising up the Missouri River. Because the captain of the vessel feared schedule delays, he failed to quarantine passengers and crew, almost all of whom were sick. As a result, the disease quickly spread to many native communities in Kansas, Missouri, and North and South Dakota. Within three months, thousands of Mandans, Arikaras, and Hidatsas had died. According to Francis Chardon, a resident of Fort Clark, North Dakota, writing in September of 1837:

All the Rees and Mandans, Men's Women's and Children, have had the disease, except for a few Old Ones, that had it in Old times, it has destroyed the seven eights of the Mandans and one half of the Rees Nation, the Rees that are encamped With the Gros Ventres have just caught it. No doubt but the one half of them will die also.[81]

Chardon's journal described the suicides of husbands and wives who

Table 4.6 Epidemics in the Great Plains, 1780–1838			
Date	Disease	Mortality	Source
seventeenth century	no direct evidence, but epidemics likely		Sundstrom, 305–43
1780s	smallpox	?	Truteau, 1:299
1832–1834	cholera and whooping cough	?	Reinhard et al., 65
1837–1838	smallpox	one-half to over three-quarters of the native population died	Chardon (1997), 124–39; Stearn, 89–90; Trimble, 82–84

did not want to outlive their relatives, all of whom had already succumbed to the dreadful illness. He also recorded the speech of 4 Bears, a Mandan warrior who, after explaining that he had always "loved the Whites," went on to exhort his people: "Listen well what I have to say, as it will be the last time you will hear Me. Think of your Wives, Children, Brothers, Sisters, Friends, and in fact all that you hold dear, are all Dead, or Dying, with their faces all rotten, caused by those dogs the whites, think of all that My friends, and rise all together and Not leave one of them alive."[82]

By the time the epidemic subsided some seven months later, more than half of the native population of the Upper Missouri had perished; mortality varied from one community to another, with some observers reporting that half to two-thirds had died, while others reported rates as high as ten out of twelve. One estimate placed the total number of dead at seventeen thousand. Among the natives of the southern Missouri region, mortality was not nearly as high, owing to a government-sponsored program of vaccination.[83]

Brazil and North America in Comparative Perspective

While the absence of densely populated, highly developed civilizations slowed, and in some cases delayed, the imposition of European colonialism in Brazil and North America, in the end, the arrival of people and institutions from the Old World produced remarkably similar consequences. As was the case in the Caribbean, Mesoamerica, and the Andes, the arrival of Europeans and their disease organisms in Brazil and North America was economically motivated, driven by competition among the European powers, all of which desired to share in the wealth of the Americas. Following close on the heels of Columbus, the Portuguese laid claim to Brazil in 1500, and during the course of the sixteenth and early seventeenth centuries, the French, British, and Dutch seized large territories in eastern North America. While the absence of a large indigenous labor force and easily extracted gold and silver deposits discouraged rapid colonization, nevertheless, contacts between natives and Europeans occurred frequently enough to provide numerous opportunities for the transfer of Old World disease organisms to Amerindian communities. And in some instances, virgin soil epidemics struck indigenous populations well in advance of the arrival of European settlers. In most regions, exploratory expeditions preceded the arrival of colonists, and while contacts between European explorers and indigenous communities were often ephemeral, even the briefest of contacts could result in the transfer of contagious illness. Once a disease organism had been introduced, the vast networks of long-established trade routes that linked native populations in all but the most remote areas ensured rapid dissemination of the illness. The introduction of epidemic disease by exploratory expeditions probably explains the abandoned villages and piles of human remains that Pilgrim colonists discovered upon landing in New England in the early 1620s, as well as the abandoned settlements that Vancouver and others encountered in the Pacific Northwest and on the Columbia Plateau during the late eighteenth century.

A comparison of mortality rates also reveals striking similarities between the history of epidemic disease in Brazil and North America and other parts of the world. While data are even more scarce for these less densely populated regions than for other areas of the Americas, it nevertheless appears that during the century following contact, virgin soil epidemics routinely resulted in mortality rates of 25 to 50 percent. Regional variations remained significant, however, and in some instances, the percentage of deaths climbed even higher, as was the case in New England in the early 1620s, where it is estimated that as much as three-quarters of the native population succumbed to a virgin soil outbreak of smallpox. And even higher mortality rates could result when several diseases converged simultaneously, as was the case in Culiacán in the 1530s, where 86 percent of the indigenous population reportedly perished as a result of dysentery, typhoid, and measles.

As was the case in both the Old World and other regions of the Americas, the violence and dislocation of military conquest followed the arrival of Europeans and contributed to rising mortality rates throughout Brazil and North America. These military operations aimed at reducing or eliminating the autonomy of indigenous communities did not cease with the end of European colonialism in the late eighteenth and early nineteenth centuries. Throughout the nineteenth century, the government of the United States continued to wage war against native societies west of the Mississippi River, and as recently as the second half of the twentieth century, the governments of Brazil, Guatemala, Ecuador, Colombia, and Peru have all sanctioned large-scale attacks against indigenous communities that they perceived posed a threat to national or international economic interests.

In spite of the striking similarities between the history of epidemics in Brazil and North America and other parts of the world, several significant differences exist. First, particularly in Brazil, the introduction of more than half a million African slaves by 1700 significantly increased opportunities for the frequent importation of smallpox and other infections. And while the connection between epidemics among Africans and native Americans is especially clear in Brazil, the presence of large African populations in other parts of the Americas, including the Caribbean and the southeastern United States, also influenced the timing and nature of disease patterns in North America.

Both economic factors and geography limited European penetration of interior regions of Brazil and North America, and as a result, vast areas remained isolated from sustained contact with colonists long after the intruders had put down roots in coastal settlements. Thus isolation played a significant role in determining disease patterns in Brazil and North America to an extent that it did not in Mesoamerica and the Andes. Native populations in the Amazonian region of Brazil enjoyed some protection from Europeans and their diseases simply as a result of their distance from centers of political and economic power along the coast. And the remote location of the Apalachee of western Florida also afforded them some measure of protection from the full impact of European colonialism, at least during the sixteenth century. The Tarahumara, residents of the southwestern section of the state of Chihuahua in northern Mexico, provide a significant case study of the benefits provided by isolation from European colonists. Throughout much of the seventeenth century, the Tarahumara sustained heavy population losses as a result of epidemics, but toward the end of the seventeenth century, they "made a conscious decision to isolate themselves from the outside world and to establish a 'region of refuge' in the inhospitable *barranca* (ravine) country of southwestern Chihuahua." As a result, while other indigenous societies in the region continued to decline and eventually disappeared altogether, by the 1940s the Tarahumaras numbered some forty thousand individuals.[84] Also significant is the fact that in at least two instances, native populations sustained heavy losses as a result of the introduction of Old World diseases, followed by periods of prolonged recovery, only to be followed later by even more severe declines. Evidence indicates that in the Southeast the size of the native population decreased between the arrival of the Vázquez de Ayllon expedition of 1526 and the arrival of de Soto in the early 1540s. Following these incursions, however, it appears that the indigenous population of the region recovered, at least in part, only to be reduced again following the arrival of missionaries at the end of the seventeenth century. A similar situation developed in the Pacific Northwest following the initial introduction of smallpox in the late 1770s: according to at least one observer, during the next decade the number of indigenous inhabitants of the region increased until recovery was cut short by the reintroduction of smallpox as well as other diseases.

Perhaps one of the most significant conclusions revealed by the study of disease patterns in Brazil and North America following the arrival of

Europeans is that even as late as the end of the nineteenth and into the twentieth century, mortality rates among indigenous populations often remained as high as those three hundred years earlier—and this at a time when mortality rates were declining significantly among populations of European and African descent in these same regions. Increasing numbers of European and African Americans reinforced the demographic, economic, and political marginalization of native Americans. Given the fact that the experience of native American peoples with epidemic disease closely resembles that of other human populations, the explanation for this disparity in matters relating to the severity of disease and mortality appears to lie in the policies of colonial powers and their successor states throughout the region.

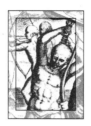

5 • New World Epidemics and European Colonialism

*S*ince epidemics can account for virtually all of the extra mortality in the sixteenth century, the principle of Occam's razor suggests that it is not necessary to assume that there were other important causes of death.

Whitmore, *Disease and Death in Early Colonial Mexico*

It is essential that scholars move away from monocausal explanations of population change to reach a broad-based understanding of decline and extinction of Native American groups after 1492.

Larsen et al.,
"Population Decline and Extinction in La Florida"

It seems to be irrevocably written in the book of fate, that the race of red men shall be wholly extirpated in the land in which they ruled the undisputed masters, til the rapacity of the Whites brought to their shores the murderous firearms, the enervating ardent spirits, and the all-destructive pestilence of the smallpox.

Stearn and Stearn,
The Effect of Smallpox on the Destiny of the American Indian

Native American and European Responses to Epidemic Disease

In light of one of the central arguments of this book, that the experience of native Americans with epidemic disease closely resembled that of people in other regions of the world, how did indigenous populations respond to the devastating waves of epidemic disease that appeared among them after 1492? How did they interpret or explain the outbreak of new diseases and the accompanying demographic catastrophe? And how did European officials and settlers respond to public health crises that surpassed in scope any they had witnessed in the Old World?

Both before and after the arrival of Europeans, native Americans made sense of illness by classifying it according to systems closely resembling the humoral model that developed in several regions of the Old World. Anthropologist Joseph Bastien, for example, argues that the Andean system was based on a cyclical theory in which health resulted from the unimpeded movement of fluids through the body. Sickness developed when the cycle was interrupted either by a blockage or by the loss of fluids.[1] Health could be restored only by reestablishing the cycle. Furthermore, Andean concepts of physiology and classification closely resembled those of the traditional European system in other ways. In form and function, the Andean three fluids of life (air, blood, and fat) correspond to the European four humors (blood, phlegm, yellow bile, and black bile); both systems also included principles of opposition with regard to the use of hot and cold categories. According to the Inca chronicler Garcilaso de la Vega, "The chill of a tertian or quartan they call *chucchu*, 'trembling,' fever is *rupa*, with a soft *r*, 'to burn.' They feared these illnesses a great deal, because of alternating extremes of hot and cold."[2]

Similar references to hot and cold classifications also exist for sixteenth-century Mexico, where Spaniards noted that natives "could explain the properties of medicinal plants by no other means."[3] Traditional Mesoamerican medical practices were based on the notion that equilibrium both within the universe and the individual was paramount to the maintenance of health and order. Within this system, physical health was achieved and maintained, in part, by the use of medicinal plants assigned hot and cold properties. Because illnesses were also classified according to hot and cold characteristics, herbal cures were prescribed in opposition. Thus for an individual suffering from a febrile disease, a medical practitioner would prescribe a cure with cold qualities. Gout and various stomach ailments, on the other hand, were classified as cold, and therefore a plant with "hot" properties was often prescribed.[4] The foregoing statements lend support to the argument that native Americans had indeed formulated classifications based on the properties of hot and cold—further evidence that a taxonomic system similar to the Old World humoral system of medicine had developed independently in the Americas.

Amidst the terror and turmoil of epidemics, the way in which native societies explained the devastation wrought by infectious disease is strikingly similar to that of Old World populations. Throughout the hemisphere after 1492, many native peoples interpreted the arrival of epidemics as divine punishment. Europeans, of course, were quick to reinforce the belief that it was their Christian god who was responsible for dispensing infectious retribution, and in fact, most colonists believed this themselves. According to the Jesuit Francisco Pries, who observed an epidemic among the native residents of Bahia, Brazil, in 1552, "Our Lord wished that these people's children, who were baptised in innocence, died in the same innocence. In this way the parents were punished but the children were saved." Farther south in Rio de Janeiro, another Jesuit "told the Indians that God was punishing them 'for the larceny they were doing in our lodgings, and for our disfavour with them. . . . ' They had the opinion that it was our captain or I who was making them die. . . . They suddenly all cried out against us, and were convinced that we had brought them this illness to make them die. They therefore plotted together to massacre us and eat us."[5]

Like the Indians of Brazil, the indigenous inhabitants of Virginia recognized that while it might be the Christian god who was punishing them, it was the Europeans themselves who "might kil and slaie whom wee would without weapons and not come neere them."[6] Ironically, the native explanation for the origins of these epidemics was partially correct: Europeans were responsible for introducing lethal pathogens into their midst, although most of the time, they did so unwittingly. Certainly it did not serve the long-term economic interests of the Spanish, Portuguese, or French to reduce the size of the indigenous population upon whom they relied for labor. However, the deliberate introduction of infectious diseases, germ warfare, as it is called today, was most certainly perpetrated by the British on a number of occasions, especially during the eighteenth century. The most infamous incident involved the British military commander Sir Jeffery Amherst, who ordered the dispatch of blankets infected with the smallpox virus to Shawnee and Delaware communities in western Pennsylvania and Ohio during a native uprising, Pontiac's Rebellion, in the summer of 1763. While the documentary record does not indicate whether or not the blankets achieved their desired result, the incident reveals the lengths to which the British were willing to go to quell the uprising. Documentation also indicates that similar events occurred in many parts of North America, and while some of these were aimed at native populations, others were not. During the Revolutionary War, for example, one aspect of British military strategy was the deliberate spread of smallpox among the troops in the army of General George Washington. And during this period, the British deliberately dispersed infected African slaves to spread smallpox among rebellious colonists in Virginia.[7]

The introduction of Old World pathogens and the subsequent arrival of Christianity forced native societies to reevaluate and reinterpret their cosmological structures. Because two sets of gods now had the potential to inflict disease, both had to be propitiated, and two distinct sets of rituals had to be followed. As a result, it became increasingly difficult for native communities and individual natives to maintain the sense of balance central to both religious systems. In the minds of native Americans, the epidemics of smallpox, measles, and other diseases that had arrived in the wake of Europeans were directly attributable to the imbalances resulting from European colonialism. Natives of the Andes, for example, had long recognized divine anger as one of several possible causes of disease. Conflicts between individuals or the breaking of taboos could also manifest themselves as sickness; however, after the conquest, divine retribution became the primary explanation for illness: "The wak'as [gods], abandoned by the people who turned to the Catholic faith, had grown hungry and vengeful toward their descendants. They sent the unfamiliar illnesses that devastated the people. . . . In order to end the illness and death, the representatives of the wak'as argued that the people had to return to the old traditions and remove the discord and disunity sown by the Spaniards.[8] "At the same time, native Americans also recognized that the god of the Christians also sent disease to punish those who refused to worship him. Thus native Americans found themselves trapped: if they ignored their *huacas* and adopted the god of the Europeans, they would suffer, and if they failed to give up their old ways, the Europeans and their Christian god would also surely punish them.

Nevertheless, evidence gathered in Spanish America clearly indicates that most natives did not give up traditional religious beliefs. In the more remote areas, where priests seldom ventured, native communities were left alone to practice their ancient rituals. In regions closer to the European sphere of influence, officials and clergy often required native participation in church activities, especially payment of the tithe. In spite of outward displays of Christian piety, however, many continued to worship their gods in secret.

Another way in which the disease experience of native Americans closely resembled that of their European counterparts was that when confronted with virgin soil epidemics, native Americans experienced the same intense feelings of terror, confusion, and despair. European observers frequently commented on the fear and hopelessness that pervaded native communities in the face of the onslaught of Europeans and their diseases. A typical example comes from a visitor to coastal Brazil in 1559 who noted the demoralizing effect of epidemics on the native population:

You can imagine how one's heart was torn with pity at seeing so many children orphaned, so many widowed, and the disease and epidemic so rife among them that it seemed like a pestilence. They were terrified and almost stunned by what was happening to them. They no longer performed their songs and dances. Everything was grief. In our aldeia there was nothing to be heard but weeping and groaning by the dying.[9]

In eastern North America, another European noted similar reactions among the Iroquois in 1679 when he wrote, "The Small Pox desolates them to such a degree that they think no longer of Meeting nor of Wars, but only of bewailing the dead, of whom there is already an immense number."[10]

In addition to terror and despair, numerous observers commented on what they perceived to be the resignation, or loss of will to live, that they claimed to have witnessed in many native communities. Diego Muñoz Camargo, a Spaniard living in Mexico during the 1580s, expressed a sentiment widely shared by many Europeans when he wrote: "They do not protect themselves from contagious illnesses; upon falling ill they are fatalistic and they permit themselves to die like beasts."[11] A German missionary noted a similar phenomenon in 1699: "The Indians die so easily that the bare look and smell of a Spaniard causes them to give up the ghost."[12] One Brazilian Jesuit complained, "Any attack of dysentery kills them; and for any small annoyance they take to eating earth or salt and die."[13] And in North America, Chardon noted a similar phenomenon during the 1837 epidemic of smallpox among the Mandan:

A young Ree that has the smallpox, told his Mother to go and dig his grave, she accordingly did so—after the grave was dug, he walked with the help of his Father to the grave, I Went Out with the Interpreter to try to pursuade him to return back to the Village—but he would not, saying for the reason that all his young friends were gone, and that he wished to follow them, towards evening he died—[14]

In the most extreme cases, observers reported that a sense of hopelessness led some individuals to commit suicide. In recounting the horrors of the Spanish conquest of Cuba, Las Casas claimed that "some began to flee into the hills while others were in such despair that they took their own lives. Men and women hanged themselves and even strung up their own children. As a direct result of the barbarity of one Spaniard (a man I knew personally) more than two hundred locals committed suicide, countless thousands in all dying this way."[15]

Statements that purport to describe a loss of will to live and suicidal behavior on the part of native Americans provide two types of information: first, a commentary on European perceptions of the emotional state of native Americans, and second, the recounting of events allegedly witnessed by these authors. Whether or not we choose to believe Las Casas's tale of mass suicides, recent medical studies clearly indicate that illness and social turmoil often produce severe depression in a significant number of people; individuals suffering from life-threatening illnesses often become depressed, even suicidal. And even once the patient has recovered, symptoms of severe depression can persist indefinitely.

In addition, individuals who survived a severe case of smallpox often faced another challenge—the devastating psychological impact of deep facial scarring. In Peru, during the smallpox epidemic of 1589, many individuals suffered from "tumors, callous excrescences or itchy scabs or very nasty pustules . . . that resulted in a monstrous ugliness in the faces and bodies."[16] According to Le Page du Pratz, a Frenchman who lived among the Natchez of Louisiana from 1718 to 1734, "The aged die in consequence of their advanced years, and the bad quality of their food; and the young, if they are not strictly watched, destroy themselves, from an abhorrence of the blotches on their skin."[17]

During the last two weeks of August 1837, Chardon noted the suicides or murder-suicides of seven individuals: the double suicides of a husband and wife, who died so as "to not Out live their relations that are dead"; a husband infected with smallpox who attacked his wife "and struck her in the head with his tomahawk, with the intent to Kill her, that she might go with him in the Other World," who later killed himself; and a young mother, whose husband had recently died of smallpox, who killed her two children and then hung herself.[18] While Las Casas may have exaggerated the numbers of suicides that took place during the Spanish conquest of the Caribbean, Chardon and others did not. The fact is that many individuals did, in fact, choose to end their lives rather than continue to submit to the harshness of life under European colonialism.

Concepts of balance and reciprocity as desirable properties applied not only to the health of individuals but also to the condition of communities and the universe beyond. Any breach of cultural norms that altered the relations of the human, natural, and spiritual realms had serious implications for society as a whole, and illness or natural disasters were often the direct consequence of such breaches. During times of crisis, in response to popular unrest and anxiety, both individuals and entire communities often sought comfort and explanation in millenarian and messianic movements. Given the extreme degree of demographic decline and social upheaval that occurred throughout the Americas in the centuries following contact with Europeans, it is not surprising that a variety of such prophetic activities flourished. Perhaps the earliest occurred in the Caribbean, the first region to experience the brunt of contact. According to a Spaniard captured by the Calusa of Florida, sometime in the early sixteenth century, Cuban natives crossed the straits between that island and the mainland, searching for the River Jordan, the waters of which were reputed to have miraculous curative powers. "So earnestly did they engage in the pursuit, that there remained not a river nor a brook in all Florida, not even lakes and ponds, in which they did not bathe."[19] Thus tales of the biblical River Jordan prompted Cuba's natives to go in search of their own healing waters.

When smallpox first appeared in Brazil in 1562, "the Indians of Bahia turned to a vision of deliverance" offered by a messianic movement called the Santidade.[20] This cult, which attracted slaves and free blacks as well as natives, promised that "their god would free them from slavery and make them masters of the white people, who would become their slaves." Despite the best efforts of Inquisition officials to eradicate the influence of this popular movement, the Santidade continued to gather strength throughout the sixteenth century.

In Peru during the same period, a messianic movement called Taki Onqoy, the dancing sickness, appeared in the southern highlands. Its leaders "preached that very soon, a pan-Andean alliance of deities would defeat the chief Christian god and kill the Spanish colonizers with disease and other calamities. Natives who wished to avoid the same fate and to enter a new, purified era of health and abundance should worship the vengeful huacas (gods) and reject all forms of cooperation with Europeans."[21] At the height of its popularity during the 1570s, Taki Onqoy posed a powerful challenge to Spanish authority in southern Peru, offering demoralized natives hope for a better future, a future in which they would regain dominance of the Andean world. By the beginning of the seventeenth century, however, divisions within native society and increased colonial control combined to undermine the power and attraction of this movement. The aggressive philosophy of Taki Onqoy was replaced by a more passive belief in the return of an Andean savior who would someday "avenge Indian society and restore the cosmos to its proper order."[22]

In response to two epidemics of smallpox that preceded the arrival of European fur traders, prophetic movements also appeared among natives of the Columbia Plateau in the Pacific Northwest during the 1770s and again between 1880 and 1881. Because these societies were not yet in regular contact with Europeans, they interpreted disease as a sign of spiritual imbalance. Prophets foretold "the imminent destruction of the world, followed by its renewal and the return of the dead—a vision deeply rooted in Plateau cosmology—[that] had an eerie cogency in a time of smallpox epidemic. Prophets held out the last and best hope for an end to the horror and a return to peace and prosperity."[23]

The Ghost Dance Movements among native peoples of the western United States during the 1870s and 1890s also arose in response to catastrophic demographic decline and the challenges posed by the expansionist actions of the government of the United States. The Ghost Dances, which coincided with the nadir of the indigenous populations of North America, "sought to assure survival as physical peoples through regaining population—bringing the dead to life—by performing the Ghost Dance ceremonies."[24] Those native societies that had experienced the most severe demographic declines were the most likely to participate in these movements, and significantly, many of these did record population increases in following years, probably owing to increased tribal solidarity and reduced emigration.[25]

Like people in all parts of the world, the most immediate response of native Americans to waves of epidemics was to try as best they could to protect themselves from the worst depredations of disease, and failing that, to attempt to cure the sick by relying on traditional treatments, especially bathing, sweating, purging, and herbal preparations, all of which were employed in various forms throughout the hemisphere. While the efficacy of Amerindian medical practices remains impossible to assess, owing in part to our lack of knowledge about many aspects of their procedures, one can assume that before the advent of modern medicine and drug therapies in the twentieth century, native American medical practices were, in general, as effective, or as ineffective, as those employed in other regions of the world.

As was also the case in the Old World, in many instances, indigenous medical practitioners and their procedures not only failed to help the patient but probably made the situation worse, ultimately hastening the demise of the individual and raising mortality rates even higher. In describing the arrival of smallpox on Hispaniola, for example, Las Casas described how the natives of that island reacted by bathing in local rivers and streams.[26] While the act of immersing oneself in water did not seal smallpox into the body of the sufferer as Las Casas and other Spaniards believed, expending the energy to reach the water probably drained what little strength many smallpox victims had and resulted in the worsening of their condition, as noted by Las Casas. When the natives of Mexico also resorted to bathing in response to an epidemic in 1531, Motolinia explained, "And it is true that they were repeatedly warned, and protected, and they were even admonished not to take baths or attempt other remedies harmful for that disease."[27]

Three centuries later, observers commented on a similar occurrence among natives of the northwest coast of the United States. In response to epidemics of malaria that first arrived in the region during the 1830s, "Indians would plunge into cold water; when chills came they retreated to sweat lodges. Sudden death followed."[28] While the connection between cold baths, sweat lodges, and malarial death rates is not clear, it is undeniable that inappropriate treatment led to the deaths of many who might eventually have recovered. During an unidentified epidemic in Brazil in 1563, one Jesuit explained "how he found the Indians trying to cure their sick by heating them on beds of leaves and branches laid over trenches of fire." After insisting that the natives remove their sick from the heat, he set about applying his own remedies, bleeding and "cutting off the corrupt skin with scissors and exposing the live flesh," both of which he claimed resulted in many cures.[29] While removing the sick from the heat of the trenches may have saved them from slowly burning to death, there is no reason to believe that cutting off affected flesh would have saved lives; in fact, contrary to the Jesuit's claim, it seems more likely that those so treated would have succumbed to secondary infections as a result of the wounds created when he cut off their skin with scissors.

In other parts of the Americas, explorers and colonists described medical procedures strikingly similar to those practiced throughout the Old World. Jacques Le Moyne, who traveled through Florida in the 1560s, noted that the Timucuans relied extensively on both bleeding and purging to cure illness.[30] Both procedures were also widely practiced among Andean societies, where regular purges "taken when they felt heavy or sluggish, more often in health than in sickness," unblocked the physiological cycle so that fluids could travel unimpeded through the body. They resorted to bleeding less frequently, but when necessary "they merely opened the vein nearest the place where they felt the pain."[31] In this way, they reasoned that bloodletting restored balance to the biological system.

In some instances, seriously ill natives resorted to extreme measures in attempting to cure themselves of the disease. According to Chardon:

A young Ree that has been sick for some time with the small pox, and being alone in his lodge, thought that it was better to die than to be in so much pain, he began to rub the scabs until blood was running all over his body, he rolled himself in the ashes, which almost burnt his soul out of his body—two days after he was perfectly well, it is a severe operation, but few are disposed to try it—however it proved beneficial to him.[32]

In this case, it is difficult to know how to explain the complete and rapid recovery of the young man; it seems just as likely that his "severe operation" could have killed him as cured him. During this same epidemic, Chardon also noted that the Rees employed more traditional procedures, including prayers to the sun and moon, the interpretation of dreams, and sacrifices.[33]

Other practices appeared silly, even outrageous, to Europeans, who did nothing to hide their contempt for indigenous medicine and its practitioners. Jean de Lery, a Frenchman who traveled through Brazil in the 1550s, clearly conveyed this sentiment when he described how the natives of the coast treated illness:

> If it happens that one of them falls sick, he points out where he hurts, whether in the arm, legs or other parts of the body, and one of his friends then sucks on this place with his mouth. Sometimes this is done by one of those charlatans among them called *pages*, that is, surgeons or physicians. . . . These quacks would have them believe that they are not only extracting their pain, but even prolonging their life.[34]

In some cases, officials and settlers took it upon themselves to experiment on desperate or unsuspecting natives. Chardon, for example, described his own attempt at curing an ailing native:

> An Indian that has been bleeding at the Nose all day, I gave him a decoction of all sorts of ingredients Mixed together, enough to Kill a Buffaloe Bull of the largest size, and stopped the effusion of Blood, the decoction of Medicine, was, a little Magnesia, peppermint, sugar lead, all Mixed together in a phial, filled with Indian grog—and the Patient snuffing up his nose three or four times— I done it out of experiement, and am content to say that it proved effectual, the Confidence that an Indian has in the Medicine of the whites, is half the cure.[35]

Chardon's contempt for the sick native and his arrogant statement regarding the placebo effect of his remedy underscores the condescending attitude of many Europeans toward native Americans.

While most Europeans regarded native American medical practices with contempt and while colonial policies clearly prohibited the continued practice of native religion, colonial officials and settlers recognized the value of the New World pharmacopoeia and strove to learn from native healers the many properties of their herbal medicines. Even Europeans who viewed native Americans as savages often had to admit their admiration for indigenous knowledge of the medicinal qualities of their native flora. Francisco Hernández, a royal physician and leader of a botanical expedition to Mexico in the 1570s, expressed a sentiment shared by many Europeans:

> I marveled, in this and in innumerable other herbs, which are nameless among us, how in the Indies, where people are so uncultured and barbaric, there are so many herbs, some with known uses and some without, but there is almost none, which is not known to them and given a particular name.[36]

The extent to which native American medical practices were changed by contact with Europeans and their diseases is not clear. While colonial policies reflected opposition to the continuation of many native American medical traditions, a chronic shortage of European-trained doctors forced colonial officials to tolerate the continued practice of native healers. Furthermore, all of the major colonial powers were concerned with abolishing specific medical practices. Fasting, for example, played an important role in both the prevention and treatment of illness before the conquest, and for that reason, officials in Spanish America tried unsuccessfully to eradicate the practice. In addition, officials of the Catholic Church urged local authorities to prohibit sacrifices of corn and other items during times of widespread illness and even to punish those who persisted in this practice. But at least one change that certainly occurred throughout the Americas was the increased use of alcohol for medical purposes. Without exception, Spanish, Portuguese, French, and British officials conspired to sell large amounts of wine and other spirits, ostensibly for medical use. According to a Spanish priest, "They would like to see all diseases treated with wine, for that is very profitable for them."[37] Although shamans and healers sometimes administered alcohol and other intoxicants to their patients, before the arrival of Europeans drunkenness unrelated to ceremonial occasions had been a serious offense in many native societies. But colonial officials not only condoned the excessive use of alcohol, they encouraged it, and as a result, alcohol poisoning, alcoholism, and related problems posed yet another threat to the health of native communities.

European responses to catastrophic epidemics in their American colonies varied. Because the scale of these outbreaks was so enormous, it was difficult for colonial governments to respond in any significant way, even when there was a desire to do so. In most instances, colonial officials lacked sufficient resources to respond, and in many cases, they also lacked the will, choosing to do nothing or waiting until it was too late. In order to deal with the health-related problems of both natives and Europeans alike, colonial officials turned to the systems of health care with which they were most familiar, establishing laws and institutions modeled on those of the colonial power. One precaution widely employed by both Spanish and Portuguese officials was the ancient practice of quarantine. And because colonial officials understood that the arrival of slave ships often meant the introduction of infectious diseases, quarantines were routinely imposed in port cities where African slaves disembarked. In Lima in 1630, the viceroy took the extraordinary precaution of ordering that all African slaves be segregated by sex and inspected by three physicians for signs of smallpox or measles before they were allowed to enter the city.[38] But most attempts to halt the spread of infectious disease were doomed to fail simply because it was impossible for colonial officials to control the movement of people throughout their jurisdictions. And at least in the highlands of Ecuador, officials largely abandoned the practice of isolating the sick during the seventeenth century.[39] English colonists, on the other hand, seldom resorted to the imposition of quarantines since they did not want to do anything that might slow the decline of native populations, thus delaying fulfillment of their goal to rid North America of its natives, clearing the way for English settlement.

Especially severe epidemics might elicit a more complex response, as was the case in Peru in 1589. The crisis posed by the epidemics of the late 1580s was so serious that in March of 1589, Viceroy Conde del Villar issued a set of specific medical instructions intended to help regional governments mitigate the effects of the disaster. On the advice of three Lima physicians, the viceroy ordered local officials throughout the Andes to quarantine all native communities in hopes of preventing the spread of disease. This measure was also intended to prevent a total breakdown of social services by forcing the healthy to remain in their homes and care for the sick. He recommended bleeding as a preventive measure and urged families to limit contact to avoid spreading infection among themselves. Those who had no one to care for them were to be brought to hospitals, public houses, and churches, where priests and local officials would provide food and medicine.[40]

The instructions also included specific dietary recommendations: the sick should be given no meat of any kind; rather, they should be fed a mixture of barley, conserves, raisins, lettuce, squash, and quinoa cooked with oil, vinegar, and sugar. They should also be provided with bread and water mixed with barley and raisins. If the patient recovered, he or she could then eat meat and drink wine and *chicha* (corn liquor). Physicians also urged patients to stay warm, to avoid sleeping on the ground, and not to drink cold water. The appearance of sores in the throat and around the eyes was regarded as a most dangerous development, and the viceroy's advisers recommended a solution of alum or copper sulfate for the throat and a bath of sugar and saffron dissolved in rose or fennel water for the eyes. Finally, the clothing of the dead was to be burned or washed many times in hot water. To what extent local officials complied with these instructions is impossible to say. Because of the considerable expense, it seems unlikely that many of these recommendations were followed. Nevertheless, the urgency and scope of these instructions suggest that the viceregal government regarded the severity of the crisis as unprecedented; they also reveal the underlying fear that the epidemics posed a long-term threat to Spanish interests throughout the viceroyalty, as indeed they did.

In Spanish America, matters affecting public health rested with local governments *(cabildos)*; these bodies wrote and enforced legislation dealing with disease and sanitation well into the twentieth century. In conjunction with wealthy citizens, cabildos often established hospitals for the care and treatment of sick natives. Hapsburg emperor Charles V founded what later became one of the largest and most important of these institutions in the Americas, the Royal Indian Hospital of Mexico City, in 1553. Similar hospitals were also established in Lima, Quito, Cartagena, Vera Cruz, Guatemala, Havana, and other urban centers. In response to a severe epidemic of plague or typhus in 1546, for example, local officials in Ecuador established the Hospital of Nuestra Señora de la Antigua. Funding for the first hospital in the northern Andes came from the sale of livestock, and a prominent cabildo member served as director. How long the hospital continued to function after 1548 is not clear, but by 1565, it had ceased to exist, probably because of insolvency.[41] In 1565, one of the first acts of a new provincial governor was to initiate construction of a hospital. At the same time, he created a charitable organization whose members were responsible for raising money and administering the new infirmary. The hospital was intended to serve both men and women, Spaniards and natives, but within a few years, it too was abandoned because of lack of support.[42] Throughout the remainder of the sixteenth century, Spanish officials attempted to establish hospitals in various regions of Ecuador, but even when funds were available, administrative corruption often diverted significant amounts of money from hospital budgets. Such a case was revealed in 1585, when the director of a local hospital refused to leave office at the end of his three-year term. Charges were eventually filed against him, and he was found guilty of stealing money from the hospital, resulting in "very bad service and little care for the poor." The ruling also noted that similar problems existed in other hospitals throughout the region.[43]

Throughout Spanish America, hospitals suffered from a chronic lack of financial support and from fiscal mismanagement. As a result, patients and their families were often forced to provide their own food, medicine, and bedding. Because conditions were poor and mortality rates high, hospitals were feared and avoided by Europeans and natives alike. Instead, many Spaniards sought out the services of unlicensed medical practitioners, apothecaries, and barber-surgeons. Most natives, on the other hand, had little contact with European medical practices and continued to rely on their own traditional systems of healing. In North America, the few hospitals that were founded during the eighteenth century were intended to serve Europeans only.

Even as late as the end of the nineteenth century, when epidemics threatened surviving native populations, the governments of the United States and Canada chose not to devote the necessary resources to preventing the spread of contagious illness or alleviating the suffering of those infected, despite demonstrated efficacies of medicines and therapies widely in place at that time. Programs to vaccinate large numbers of Indians, initiated in 1801 by President Thomas Jefferson, were never adequately funded. As a result, major outbreaks of smallpox continued to decimate native societies well into the twentieth century, while white citizens were protected. Furthermore, because the smallpox vaccine lost its efficacy with age, it was often rendered useless by the time it arrived in native communities. In some instances, however, natives performed their own inoculations, as was the case at Fort Clark in 1837, when a man inoculated his child "by cutting two small pieces of flesh out of his arms, and two on the belly—and then takeing a Scab from one, that was getting well of the disease, and rubbing it on the wounded part, three days after, it took effect and the child is perfectly well."[44] In both the United States and Canada, the government agencies that dealt with the affairs of native populations were woefully underfunded and the money available for emergency supplies of food, medicines, and bedding was insufficient or nonexistent.

Just as the actions of colonial governments varied, so too did the responses of individual Europeans. While many remained unaware of or chose to ignore the suffering of native communities during times of epidemics, others pitched in, providing food, clothing, and nursing services. In response to the smallpox epidemic that struck New England during the 1630s, some English colonists, "seeing their woefull and sadd condition, and hearing their pitifull cries and lamentations, they had compassion of them, and dayly fetched them wood and water, and made them fires, gott them victualls whilst they lived, and buried them when they dyed."[45] More than two centuries later, administrators from the Bureau of Indian Affairs also noted that during the smallpox epidemic of 1898–1899, many whites risked their own lives in order to tend to the needs of hundreds of sick and dying Pueblo. But many others, including a number of bureau employees, abandoned their native charges in their time of need.[46]

In most cases, before the twentieth century, basic nursing care combined with adequate food, water, and clean bedding were the most effective measures available in both the Old World and the New. But Europeans repeatedly noted that because so many individuals were stricken simultaneously, it was often impossible to provide even the most fundamental care. In his *History of Plymouth Plantation*, William Bradford described the pitiful state of one native community outside a Dutch trading post during the 1630s:

> The condition of this people was so lamentable, and they fell downe so generally of this diseas [smallpox], as they were (in the end) not able to help one another; no, not to make a fire, nor to fetch a little water to drink, nor any to burie the dead; but would strivie as long as they could, and when they could procure no other means to make fire, they would burn the woden trays and dishes they ate their meate in, and their very bows and arrowes; and some would crawle out on all foure to gett a litle water, and some times dye by the way, and not be able to gett in agine.[47]

The difference that adequate nursing care can make is clearly illustrated by a recent study that compared rates of mortality among Hopi communities in New Mexico during an epidemic of smallpox in 1898–1899. According to records maintained by the Bureau of Indian Affairs, among a population of 421 Hopi who accepted nursing care, 24 persons died; this compared to 163 deaths among the 220 Hopi who refused care. Mortality rates of 6 and 74 percent for these two populations clearly demonstrate the significant difference that basic care could make.[48]

The responses of native Americans to the onslaught of virgin soil epidemics that struck them in the wake of European expansion closely resembled the responses of peoples in the Old World under similar circumstances. Just as the indigenous populations of the Americas suffered mortality rates similar to those experienced by Old World populations, they also responded to the challenges posed by epidemic disease in a similar fashion. The emotions experienced, the explanations offered, and the treatments adopted by native Americans all demonstrate the universal nature of the human response to epidemic disease. In spite of these striking similarities, however, one significant difference exists. If the severe labor shortages that resulted from the bubonic plague epidemics of the fourteenth century ultimately benefited Western Europeans by leading to higher wages, the development of new technologies, and the adoption of elite strategies to limit family size by the poor, why did similar developments fail to materialize in the Americas? Why did demographic decline fail to improve the social and economic situation of native Americans?

The Impact of European Colonialism

Studies of the long-term demographic impact of epidemics have often noted a strong correlation between the degree of elite control over the people and natural resources of a region and the recovery or failure to recover of both human populations and economies. Watts has argued that following severe epidemics, the degree of demographic and economic recovery was most affected by "the institutional framework and mindset of the governing classes." As examples, he cited the cases of Sicily and Tuscany following the bubonic plague epidemics of the fourteenth century, noting that in the former, political rivalries between ruling elites resulted in a weaker authoritarian structure that facilitated the creation of new economic strategies for the region's poor in the wake of population decline, while in Tuscany, elite control remained highly centralized and as a result, "tax burdens and labor requirements imposed on ordinary people prevented them from rising above the poverty level."[49] In chapter 1, similar developments were noted in the discussion of bubonic plague epidemics in Europe, where the public health measures implemented by local authorities following the Black Death hastened the disappearance of plague from much of the region, while the failure of their counterparts in the Middle East to adopt similar strategies resulted in frequent recurrences that reduced populations and retarded economic development until the middle of the nineteenth century. Because elite control appears to play such a significant role in the ability of societies to recover from demographic disaster, an examination of the colonial policies of Spain, Portugal, Britain, and France reveals much about the long-term impact of disease on Amerindian populations.

Motives and Methods: Military Conquest

The colonial policies of each of the four major European powers reflected both the cultural biases and economic and political motivations of each. Of the four, Spain was the only colonial power to conquer densely populated agricultural societies and the only one to enjoy immediate access to valuable mineral resources. In response to these factors, Spain developed the most institutionalized and complex set of policies for dealing with its indigenous subjects. From the beginning, Spain's interest in its American territories was the conquest of native populations, the collection of tribute, and the extraction of mineral wealth, an arduous task to be carried out by a seemingly infinite supply of indigenous labor. But before Spanish colonists and adventurers could begin profiting from the enormous wealth of the Americas, they first had to subdue indigenous populations. On the islands of the Caribbean and later on the mainland, Spanish armies, usually accompanied by large numbers of native allies, fought military campaigns that claimed tens of thousands of lives and destroyed the material

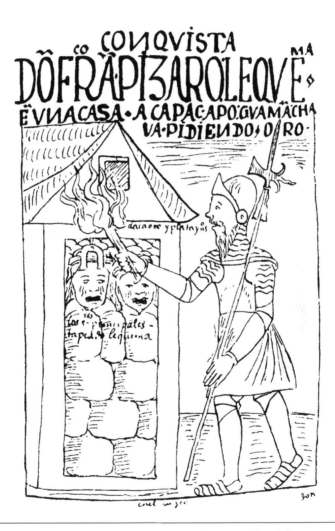

Fig. 14. *The death of Capac Apo Guaman Chava, uncle of the Inca chronicler Guaman Poma. (Guaman Poma,* Nueva corónica, *1613)*

prosperity of countless indigenous societies. Although specific estimates are difficult to come by owing mostly to a lack of documentation from these earliest years of the conquest, sufficient information can be culled from the chronicles of various regions to give some indication of the severity and extent of the violence. Newson, for example, estimated that during the conquest of Honduras in the 1530s, between 30,000 and 50,000 indigenous residents were killed in defending their territory against Spanish armies.[50] During the brief space of several hours at Cajamarca in 1532, more than 2000 natives lost their lives in the fighting that led to the Spanish capture of the Inca emperor Atahualpa.[51] But such specific estimates are rare; more often one is left to infer the extent of the violence through commentaries on the size of native armies and the duration of military engagements. During the conquest of Guatemala from 1524 to 1530, for example, the Spanish and their native allies fought seven major battles against local armies that numbered between 5000 and 10,000 warriors. And while the chroniclers offer no estimates of mortality, ultimately this warfare resulted in the defeat of indigenous forces and the deaths of thousands of Maya.[52] Similarly, the Mixton War, which erupted in northern Mexico in 1541 and pitted local societies against a Spanish army of several hundred supported by 30,000 native allies from central Mexico, resulted in the enslavement of thousands of natives and the deaths of many thousands more.[53]

In his third letter to King Charles V of Spain, Cortés made clear the dilemma he and many other conquerors faced: "I knew not what means to adopt to relieve our dangers and hardships, and to avoid utterly destroying them and their city, which was the most beautiful thing in the world."[54] Cortes's admiration for the cultural achievements of the Mexica was clearly reflected in many of his writings, but in the end, the conqueror of Mexico was not able to prevent the destruction of Tenochtitlán as fighting to secure the capital proceeded systematically from one neighborhood to the next. According to Cortes's description of the battle for one sector of the city, "The fight between us and our enemies was very stubborn, but finally we won that whole quarter, and, such was the slaughter committed upon our enemies, that between killed and wounded there were more than twelve thousand."[55] And when the siege of the city finally ended, the conqueror, Bernal Díaz del Castillo, described houses, streets, and canals full of the bodies of dead Mexica.[56] While the struggle for control of Tenochtitlán was perhaps the largest single conflict the Spanish faced in the Americas, throughout their empire, similar wars were waged on smaller, less centralized societies. And the end result was always the same—the loss of thousands of lives and the erosion of traditional economic and political infrastructures.

But military campaigns were not the only drain on native populations

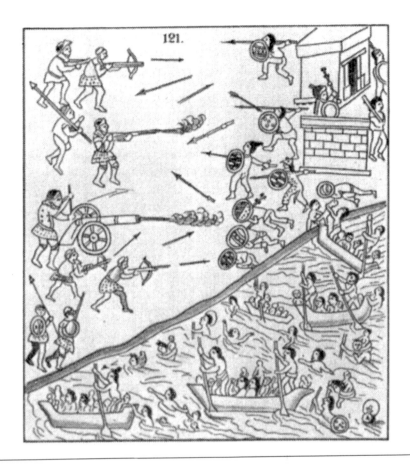

Fig. 15. *The Spanish conquest of Tenochtitlán by a native artist. (Florentine Codex, 1590)*

during the early years of the conquest, as most military commanders launched exploratory expeditions as soon as they had secured their bases of operation. A typical example comes from Ecuador, where less than two years after the founding of the city of Quito, the town council ordered that no more natives be taken out of the area "because this province has few Indians." This decree was in part a response to a letter from Francisco Pizarro stating his concern that the native population was rapidly declining. Between 1534 and 1580, at least twenty-nine major expeditions, including approximately fifty thousand native men and women, left Quito. Few ever returned. Some died in battles; many more died of starvation and disease. Still others were sold into slavery to the north in New Granada.[57]

European seizure of native lands was another important factor in the failure of native societies to recover fully following their incorporation into the Spanish empire. For within a generation, much of the most productive agricultural properties had been confiscated by Spanish colonists. While *encomiendas* (a grant of native tribute and labor conferred by the Spanish crown on individual Spaniards) did not confer legal title to land, in practice many *encomenderos* seized property from the natives under their control. In many instances, conquerors staked legal claims to whatever lands they deemed most desirable, usually those that were close to their encomienda populations. In many instances, Spaniards argued that land was vacant, whether or not in fact it was. They were aided in these efforts by the rapid decline in the number of natives, opening up more land for Spanish occupation. The speed with which the alienation of native lands occurred was indeed remarkable. In Ecuador, for example, records indicate that only seven months after the initial arrival of Spaniards in the Quito area, most of the best, most accessible lands had already been distributed and that they were beginning to run short of land to distribute to the steady stream of European newcomers who continued to arrive.[58] Many natives were also forced to sell their lands in order to cover tribute obligations. The alienation of native lands worsened over time as many more Spaniards and their descendents laid claim to ever-increasing amounts of property. As a result of both immigration and natural increase, the white population of Spanish America had grown to over five hundred thousand by 1650, with the majority of those individuals concentrated in Mexico and Peru.[59] As a result, by the eighteenth century, when the native populations of many areas finally began to increase, insufficient land remained under indigenous control. The alienation of native lands undermined the indigenous economy and ultimately forced many natives onto Spanish-owned haciendas and ranches.

While Spain's colonial policies emphasized the conquest of native peoples, the collection of tribute, and the extraction of mineral wealth, the policies pursued by its Iberian neighbor, Portugal, differed both in focus and extent. Because the Portuguese government chose to concentrate its resources and energies on developing its possessions in Africa and the Far East, the colonization of Brazil proceeded more slowly and along a different path than that of Spanish America. Unlike Spanish monarchs, who moved quickly to consolidate control over newly discovered territories and to retain direct control over the governing of their colonies, the government of Portugal viewed its American colony as secondary in importance to its holdings in the east, and as a result, it was willing to entrust its development to individuals and families rather than taking a more direct role in the process of colonization. Following its discovery by Cabral in 1500, Brazil was largely ignored by the Portuguese crown until 1532, when King João III awarded a series of hereditary captaincies to individuals empowered to promote settlement and export local resources. Brazil's lack of readily exploitable mineral deposits also slowed efforts at colonization, at least until gold was discovered at the end of the seventeenth century. A dwindling supply of native labor and the lack of easily exploited natural resources explain, in part, the slow growth of Brazil's white population, from twenty-five thousand in 1600 to a hundred thousand a century later. Because of the rapid decline of Brazil's native population and because the colonial government was not interested in creating and funding a large bureaucracy, the Portuguese chose to tax the goods traded by native communities rather than to collect a head tax, as did the government of Spain.

During the sixteenth century, the export of brazilwood and sugar constituted the foundations of the colonial economy, and as a result, demand for indigenous labor was strong. Because Brazil's natives had no tradition of large-scale organized labor, most Amerindians resisted their forced induction into the colonial workforce. In response, Portuguese colonists resorted to military campaigns and slave raiding, first among coastal populations and later among indigenous residents of the interior. These raids provoked further clashes, resulting in many deaths, especially among natives, who proved ill equipped when confronted with Portuguese firearms and swords.

When indigenous populations resisted colonial control, the Portuguese pursued wars of extinction against recalcitrant communities. Such was the case in the 1560s, when Brazil's governor, Mem da Sa, waged a "just" war against the Caete, who lived along Brazil's north-central coast, for their killing of a Portuguese bishop, shipwrecked in the area in 1556. Colonists seized upon the governor's campaign against the Caete as an excuse to enslave "any Indians of any tribe on the grounds that they might be Caete."[60] As a result, within a period of several weeks, much of the native population of the region had either been killed or enslaved. Even natives who resided in Jesuit missions were not immune to the violence, as evidenced by a sharp decline in the number of native inhabitants in four local missions, from 12,000 to 1000, during this period.[61] More than a decade later, retribution for the killing of this same bishop and other members of his party was cited as justification for a military campaign against the natives of a neighboring area, more than 1600 of whom were killed while another 4000 were captured and enslaved.[62] During the last quarter of the sixteenth century, the Portuguese launched a series of attacks against the Portiguars, who had been allied with French traders since the 1550s. During the 1570s and 1580s, the Portiguars won several significant battles against the Portuguese, but by 1601, after much bloodshed on both sides, the two parties agreed to a truce.[63]

Throughout the colonial period, the Portuguese were effectively able to exploit long-standing rivalries between native communities to their own advantage. Such was the case in the early 1600s, following the submission of the Portiguars, when the Portuguese used their recently vanquished enemies to pursue a war of conquest against the nomadic Aimore. The Aimore were inhabitants of the coastal forests around Porto Seguro and Ilheus in central Brazil, who had attacked Portuguese settlers. Ultimately the Portiguars defeated the Aimore, killing many and settling on the territory of their traditional enemies.[64] By the early seventeenth century, having successfully subdued or exterminated most coastal populations, the Portuguese turned their attention to the conquest of the indigenous inhabitants of Brazil's vast interior. And during the next two centuries, warfare and slave raiding resulted in the same devastation inland that had occurred along the Atlantic seaboard.

Like Portugal, France also lacked the resources and the will to assume primary responsibility for the colonization of its American possessions. As a result, the government of France entrusted the settlement and exploitation of its newly acquired territories both to individuals and commercial companies. Between 1599 and 1789, the crown granted at least seventy-five charters aimed at encouraging private investors to undertake the colonization of various regions of the Americas. These charters, issued to companies as well as individuals, granted wide-ranging powers and privileges, including the ownership of vast tracts of land, trade monopolies, and administrative authority. By the 1660s, however, private efforts at colonization had foundered and the crown was forced to assume responsibility for the governing of its American territories.

Unlike Spain's Council of the Indies, which oversaw all aspects of colonial policy, France had no central government office to deal solely with colonial affairs; rather, all issues pertaining to colonial matters were the purview of the Ministry of the Marine. Not only was French bureaucratic control over its American colonies more lax than that of its Iberian counterparts, its economic control was more relaxed as well. Because Canada lacked large indigenous populations and easily exploitable resources, throughout the colonial period, France received no fiscal profits from Canada and in fact was forced to subsidize its largest colony.[65]

During the seventeenth and eighteenth centuries, relatively few Frenchmen and even fewer Frenchwomen decided to emigrate to Canada: in 1663, only 2200 French settlers inhabited the region; by 1700 that number had swelled to 15,000; and by 1759, it had grown to 70,000, although much of the latter growth was due to natural increase rather than to immigration.[66] Because Canada attracted relatively few settlers, of necessity, French colonial policy was based on the idea of consent rather than conquest. The language employed in drafting the commission that formalized French settlement of Canada in 1603 illustrated the French emphasis on alliances and peaceful negotiations with indigenous leaders. The charter urged the leader of the expedition, Lord De Monts, "to negotiate and develop peace, alliance and confederation, good friendship, connections and communication with said people and their princes. . . . To maintain, respect, and carefully observe the treaties and alliances you have agreed upon with them."[67] Unlike the Spanish, Portuguese, and English, the French often sought to win the support and approval of their indigenous subjects before resorting to violence. While clearly based on relations of inequality, these alliances helped the French to legitimize their presence in the New World.

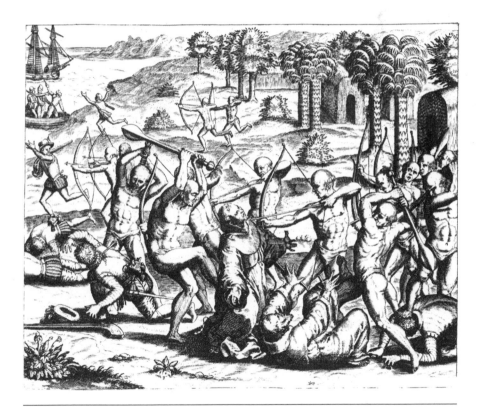

Fig. 16. *Natives of Cumana, Brazil, killing their priests. (Engraving by Theodore de Bry, 1596)*

The colonial economy of Canada rested on the export of furs provided by the region's indigenous inhabitants to French traders who traveled throughout the vast territory, exchanging manufactured goods and alcohol for beaver pelts. Because so few Europeans chose to emigrate to Canada during the seventeenth and eighteenth centuries, the French presence in North America was always tenuous. In the thousands of miles of territory that became New France, several dozen trading posts were all that constituted the French presence in the region. According to historian William Nester, the French "did not 'conquer' New France; they merely paid very high tolls to the Indians for the privelege of exploiting it."[68] By 1685, some eight hundred French traders lived and worked in the area east of the Mississippi.[69] Because of their isolation, it is not surprising that in order to ensure their own survival, traders often chose to marry indigenous women, thereby gaining access to the kin networks of their wives. According to one scholar, "French authority over North America rested on the hegemony of these kin networks."[70]

While French colonial policy emphasized alliances and consent, it also sanctioned the use of force when necessary. But rather than engage in direct military conflicts with the region's indigenous inhabitants, a strategy that would have rendered France's colonial venture not only costly but untenable, the French effectively exploited hostilities between indigenous groups. This tactic pitted native communities against each other and had the advantage of freeing France from the costly obligation of supporting a large military force in Canada; in addition, it also minimized the loss of French lives because colonial policies encouraged natives to fight each other rather than French colonists.

This strategy of relying on indigenous surrogates to fight their battles proved especially effective when it came to the ongoing struggle between England and France, a struggle that was played out in both Europe and North America in a series of five wars fought between 1627 and 1763. Owing to a number of violent encounters with the French early in the seventeenth century, the Iroquois became their most formidable enemies and eventually staunch allies of the British. For their part, the French enjoyed the support of the Hurons, Algonquians, and other native peoples of the Saint Lawrence Valley. By the 1640s, violent struggles for control of territory erupted in a series of "beaver wars," resulting in the destruction of many villages by Iroquois war parties. According to historian William Nester, "The Iroquois virtually exterminated the Huron by 1649, the Petun by 1650, the Neutrals by 1651, the Erie by 1657, and the Susquehannock by 1660."[71] Throughout this period, the Iroquois also raided French settlements, killing and capturing many colonists. But epidemics of smallpox and measles combined with incessant warfare had taken their toll, and by the end of the seventeenth century, the Iroquois and French had agreed to end the conflict.[72]

The desire for wealth also impelled the English to colonize North America. But the search for the Northwest Passage to Asia, the hunt for precious metals, and daring raids on Spanish treasure fleets soon gave way to the less exciting but ultimately more productive strategies of exporting both people and manufactured goods to England's small but expanding settlements in the Americas. Of all the European nations with an interest in colonizing North America, the English best understood the growing importance of international trade, and as a result, they occupied their colonial possessions with an eye to expanding commercial opportunities for English products.

In marked contrast to the French policy of consent, English colonial policies were designed to marginalize, isolate, and ultimately exterminate native populations. Unlike the Spanish and Portuguese, who instituted policies designed to exploit native labor and Christianize indigenous populations, and the French, who were willing to work with and live alongside native peoples, English settlers were motivated by a desire for control of native lands. In marked contrast to many Spanish and Portuguese immigrants, who planned to stay in the Americas only long enough to make their fortunes and return to their homeland, English colonists arrived in the New World with the avowed intention of remaining. According to English common law, occupation of land through the construction of a house established legal title to that property.[73] Unlike the other three colonial powers, whose laws concerning property ownership all involved written documentation in order to confer legal title, for the English, the key lay in demonstrating improvements to the land. And since, in the eyes of the English, native communities had failed to improve their lands, either through construction of permanent dwellings, agricultural operations of sufficient scale, or animal husbandry, these lands could justifiably be claimed by those who would work to improve them by "building fences, planting gardens, constructing houses—the English signs of possession."[74] Thus the occupation of native lands quickly became the focus of English colonial activity. And the most effective way to ensure unfettered access to those lands was by the forcible removal of all indigenous inhabitants. The English were aided in this endeavor by their racist attitudes toward Amerindians. Perhaps more than any other European nation, the English viewed native Americans as savages, unworthy of consideration and incapable of redemption. According to one colonial official, "It is infinitely better to have no heathen among us, who were at best as thorns in our sides, than to be at peace and league with them."[75] And if the indigenous inhabitants of the

Americas did not deserve humane treatment, therefore they could justifiably be relegated to the farthest edges of England's American world. That the English, like the French, also chose not to create an institution charged specifically with the governing of their American colonies meant that without a central body to make and enforce colonial policies, English settlers operated in a world largely without reference to moral authority, at least in matters concerning the treatment of natives. The absence of a powerful, official presence allowed colonists to act with impunity when dealing with indigenous peoples.

Like the French, Dutch, and Portuguese, the English also chose to manage their colonies through trading companies, in this case, the two most important being the Virginia Company of Plymouth, whose territory extended from Maine to the Potomac River, and the Virginia Company of London, which controlled lands extending from Cape Fear to the Hudson River. Reflecting the geographic division of these two commercial entities, English settlement of North America had two foci: the first in Virginia, beginning in the 1580s, and the second in New England, from the 1620s on. In both regions, tensions between settlers and natives developed almost immediately and warfare between the two groups erupted periodically throughout eastern North America during the seventeenth and eighteenth centuries. Ultimately, violence between English colonists and natives proved extremely costly in human lives lost on both sides. In Virginia, between 1616 and 1620, fighting broke out between English settlers and local natives, resulting in the destruction of villages and food supplies and the slaughter of populations. Then in 1622, the Pamunkey, the largest native confederation in the mid-Atlantic region, killed some four hundred English settlers in a surprise raid; again, in 1644, natives in Virginia killed five hundred colonists. As a result, the governor of Virginia ordered the systematic destruction of numerous indigenous villages and their inhabitants.[76] Survivors were forced to abandon their lands and relocate to interior regions of Virginia and the Carolinas. But Virginia was not the only region to experience prolonged violence between natives and colonists. In Connecticut in 1637, English settlers went to war against the Pequots, eventually destroying their settlement and killing more than five hundred individuals, and in Massachusetts in 1645, English colonists nearly wiped out the Narragansetts.[77] English massacres of indigenous populations served not only to clear the land for English occupation; they also served as a brutal example to neighboring societies not to oppose the growing power of English settlers.

But the most destructive war between England and its native subjects was fought in the 1670s in New England. Between 1675 and 1676, King Philips War, as it came to be known, claimed the lives of more than three thousand natives and some one thousand colonists.[78] In addition to these casualties, many natives were sold into slavery in the West Indies, while others were forced to resettle in western New York.[79] At the same time, in Virginia, three hundred colonists and hundreds of natives were killed in fighting that erupted over an attack launched by English settlers against a Susquehannock village. Wrangling between Virginia's Governor Berkeley and local leader Francis Bacon eventually resulted in fighting between the two factions. Berkeley's troops defeated both Bacon and the natives with the result that "the Indian survivors ceded most of Virginia to the English and agreed to settle on reservations.[80]

Throughout the eighteenth century, England's colonial policy centered on the creation of a frontier separating natives from rapidly growing numbers of colonists. In fact, by 1750, English North America boasted a white population of over 1 million.[81] But this policy proved impossible to enforce as English settlers repeatedly overran native lands, either forcing the indigenous population to relocate to less desirable lands or killing them outright. By the 1780s, England's policies of isolating and exterminating native populations had been adopted by the government of the newly independent United States, and especially during the nineteenth century, the notion of Manifest Destiny and transcontinental expansion justified numerous military campaigns aimed at removing indigenous inhabitants from lands coveted by white settlers. Once again, it is impossible to estimate the numbers of natives who perished in military clashes with U.S. troops and settlers, but they certainly numbered in the many thousands.

In addition to epidemic disease, violence and military conquest played a major role in the demographic decline of native American populations throughout the hemisphere after 1492. Beginning at the end of the fifteenth century and continuing well into the twentieth, organized campaigns of violence against native populations were sanctioned first by European colonial powers and later by newly independent governments throughout the hemisphere. Any attempt to understand the delayed population recovery (or failed recovery) of native American populations must take this important factor into account.

Indigenous Slavery

Warfare was not the only form of violence that accelerated the decline of native American populations. Throughout the New World, European colonial powers imposed the institution of chattel slavery, and ultimately, this form of violence proved at least as destructive as military confrontations. Spanish law permitted the enslavement of peoples who refused to submit to royal authority, *indios de guerra*, or who practiced pagan rituals such as cannibalism; it also permitted Spaniards to acquire

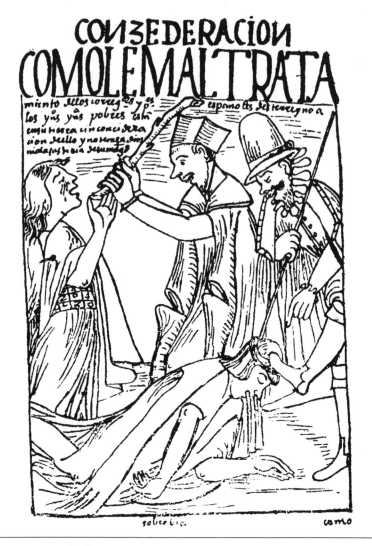

Fig. 17. *Spaniards abusing Peruvian natives. (Guaman Poma,* Nueva corónica, *1613)*

indigenous slaves from their Amerindian owners, *indios de rescate.* In some areas of Spanish America during the sixteenth century, the trade in indigenous slaves was the easiest and most lucrative economic activity available to many colonists. One area that was especially hard hit by the traffic in native slaves was Central America. Beginning in 1515, Spanish slavers regularly staged raids along the Atlantic coast, and as early as 1525, the Bay Islands of Honduras had been completely depopulated.

During the height of this trade in the 1530s, some fifteen to twenty ships devoted themselves entirely to the transfer of indigenous slaves from one port to another. Estimates of the number of Amerindians sold into slavery from Honduras and Nicaragua alone range from two hundred thousand to five hundred thousand between 1515 and 1548, when the Spanish governor finally outlawed the practice. The majority of those enslaved were exported to the Caribbean, Panama, and later Peru.[82] And while colonial observers often noted the devastating impact of epidemic disease on the native peoples of Central America, it is significant that they placed the greatest blame for population loss on the slave trade that, according to one royal official in Nicaragua, had led to the deaths of one-third of the native population.[83]

In spite of the fact that Spanish law allowed slavery to exist under specific circumstances, in general, Spain discouraged the practice, first with the promulgation of the Laws of Burgos in 1512, which attempted to regulate Spanish treatment of Amerindians, and later through the New Laws of 1542, which outlawed the enslavement of indigenous peoples except under unusual circumstances. In addition to moral arguments against slavery, and because indigenous slaves did not pay tribute, Spanish officials were also concerned about declining royal revenues. As growing numbers of Spanish colonists arrived after 1492, demand for Amerindian workers increased rapidly. Thus it was in the economic interests of Spanish officials and settlers to preserve as much of the native population as possible. Nevertheless, especially during periods of military conquest, enslavement of indigenous peoples was widespread throughout the Spanish empire.

Both Spain and Portugal permitted the enslavement of native populations that resisted conquest, but indigenous slavery in Portuguese America differed both in terms of its scale and scope. Portugal's greater tolerance for indigenous slavery derived from the fact that because Brazil's Amerindian societies were smaller and less developed than those of Spain's two most important colonies, Mexico and Peru, officials and settlers viewed force as the only way to ensure adequate supplies of native labor. And because Brazil lacked easily exploitable mineral deposits, slaving was often the only incentive to attract and retain Portuguese settlers. Like the Spanish, Portuguese law permitted the enslavement of natives who resisted conquest, but in most cases, Portuguese settlers viewed this as a technicality to be ignored. The notion that Brazil's indigenous inhabitants were inferior to Europeans and therefore "natural slaves" further served to reinforce the practice.[84]

An indication that concern for the welfare of the Portuguese government's indigenous subjects was not a top priority is the fact that the first royal edict dealing explicitly with Amerindian affairs was not promulgated until 1548, almost fifty years after Portugal first laid claim to Brazil. And while this document declared that conversion of the indigenous population was to be the major focus of colonial policy, it "also permitted the issue of slaving licenses to trustworthy persons in time of need, and it ordered wars on hostile tribes and the enslavement of captives in such wars."[85] As a result of this confusing and often ambiguous policy, a lucrative trade in indigenous slaves had developed by the 1550s. In a half-hearted attempt to reduce the worst depredations of indigenous slavery, in 1570, King Sebastiao issued an edict proclaiming that natives "may on no account and in no way be enslaved."[86] But once again, the ambiguous language of the law provided for enough exceptions, including "just wars," that the trade continued to flourish.

By the 1560s, some 40,000 native slaves toiled in the sugarcane fields of Bahia alone, and raiding expeditions throughout that region captured another 2000 to 3000 annually.[87] One expedition, launched in 1572 into the interior of Porto Seguro, ended in the enslavement of the Tupiguen, a community of some 7000 individuals. In some instances, slaving expeditions could last for years. During the 1590s around São Paulo, slaving expeditions destroyed 300 villages and killed or enslaved 30,000.[88] Throughout the seventeenth and eighteenth centuries, slave raiding was widespread, even following the official abolition of indigenous slavery in 1748.

Both the French and English permitted the enslavement of native populations, and especially during the seventeenth and early eighteenth centuries, the institution was widely practiced and produced devastating demographic consequences. In Canada, many of the slaves sold or traded to French colonists were captured as the result of raids between indigenous groups. But because large-scale agricultural production was not of economic significance, slave labor had little value. Thus in French North America, with the exceptions of Louisiana and the sugar islands of the Caribbean, where dwindling indigenous populations were enslaved by settlers and officials alike, most native slaves served as status symbols rather than valuable economic producers.[89]

Not so in parts of English North America, however. While South Carolina was the only English colony to make extensive use of indigenous slave labor, the enslavement of native populations occurred in every region from northern New England through the mid-Atlantic and into the South. Not only did English colonists retain native slaves for their own use, but a lucrative slave trade developed, resulting in the shipment of many natives to the Caribbean sugar islands and other distant regions, where the demand for labor was strong. The tensions between England's official colonial policy and the demands of North American colonists provide a revealing illustration of the difficulties inherent in trying to regulate a practice that served to benefit many colonists. In 1671, the governor of South Carolina outlawed the enslavement of that region's native inhabitants, but within less than a decade, new legislation had loosened restrictions on the trade in indigenous slaves. Once again, in 1687, English colonial officials attempted to abolish the enslavement of natives, but this attempt too ended in failure because of settler resistance, and the practice continued unabated. Finally, in 1690, the legislature of South Carolina passed further regulations, in effect legitimating the slave trade.[90]

By the beginning of the eighteenth century, having largely exhausted the local supply of natives, colonists in South Carolina were raiding into northern Florida in search of slaves. One expedition in 1704, for example, resulted in the capture of some 1300 Apalachees.[91] Between 1711 and 1712, hostilities between natives and settlers in North Carolina ignited the Tuscarora War, resulting in the deaths of many natives and the enslavement of countless others. Similar incidents of hostilities between natives and colonists resulted in the Yemassee War, fought between 1715 and 1717 in South Carolina. In both instances, military confrontations served as an excuse for extensive slave raiding. Ultimately, the catastrophic decline of the native population of South Carolina as a result of the Tuscarora and Yemassee Wars, epidemic disease, and declining birth rates resulted in steadily declining numbers of indigenous slaves. For example, between 1715 and 1725, the number of native slaves in one South Carolina parish declined from approximately ninety to fifty individuals.[92]

What occurred in South Carolina is not atypical of what happened in many regions of the New World after 1492. Wherever Europeans introduced the institution of chattel slavery, the results were uniformly the same—plummeting native populations. In combination with virgin soil epidemics and warfare, the institution of indigenous slavery placed yet another stressor on conquered populations, accelerating both their demographic decline and the erosion of their traditional economic, cultural, and political foundations.

Indigenous Labor and Migration

In addition to the stresses associated with the widespread violence of war and slavery, native American societies faced the added pressures of harsh labor regimes and, in many instances, forced migrations that proved highly disruptive to demographic recovery. From the sixteenth century to the twentieth, resettlement inevitably meant removal to less productive, less accessible lands. And even when migration was undertaken voluntarily, in search of more lucrative employment, for example, it often meant abandoning both property and culture.

Access to and control of native labor is a key to understanding the colonial policies of Spain and to a lesser extent those of Portugal, France, and England. Of the four major colonial powers, Spain developed the most complex set of regulations designed to exploit native labor most efficiently. Spanish policies did not remain static; rather, they changed over time in response to the decline of indigenous populations and changes in the economic structure of the empire itself. As early as 1498, Columbus instituted a system of labor control on the island of Hispaniola in response to Spanish demands for workers and personal servants. Based on the long-established Iberian practice of rewarding successful military commanders with vassals from conquered territories, Columbus awarded encomiendas to his friends and supporters. Against the wishes of Spanish monarchs, who opposed the distribution of encomiendas in the Americas, the conquerors and governors who followed Columbus continued this practice, with the result that by the end of the sixteenth century, hundreds of grants, ranging in size from fewer than one hundred natives to more than one hundred thousand in the case of Cortés, had been made throughout Spanish-controlled territory. The recipients of these grants, encomenderos, soon constituted the new elite of Spain's American colonies. The institution of encomienda placed heavy burdens on native communities for tribute payments and labor quotas. While tribute and labor obligations varied regionally, in general, all adult males were required to serve a turn on a rotating basis, working on Spanish-owned farms, in mines, or on public works projects. During the first half of the sixteenth century, tribute payments were assessed in goods, many of which were costly and not readily available to natives. But by the beginning of the seventeenth century and for the remainder of the colonial period, most natives paid their tribute in currency. Concurrently, the Spanish crown reasserted its control over encomiendas throughout much of its American territory, and especially after 1600, increasing numbers of these grants reverted to royal control. But colonists still relied upon the labor of native workers, and in response to their growing needs, new systems based on rotating labor drafts developed. The *repartimiento*, as it was known in Mexico and Central America, and its Andean equivalent, the *mita*, provided colonial officials and landowners with a steady supply of workers forced to toil on public works projects, in mines, on large agricultural estates, or in primitive textile factories in exchange for extremely low wages.

By the beginning of the seventeenth century, following the consolidation of Spanish control over most of Mexico, Central America, and

South America, colonial policy reflected a concern for the survival, if not the welfare, of native subjects. And the forms of labor that developed in each region were determined in large measure by local economic activities, primarily ranching, mining, agriculture, and textile production. In frontier regions of northern Mexico and southern South America, where colonists often faced bellicose, nomadic populations, slave raids continued at least until the end of the seventeenth century. In areas such as central Mexico and Peru, where larger, sedentary populations resided, coercive labor drafts and, in some areas, free wage labor, predominated.

One of the most significant consequences of the development of these varied labor systems was the forced and voluntary migration of a significant percentage of the native population. A variety of factors drove native migration throughout the colonial period: Many natives and their families moved away to escape onerous tribute and labor obligations; others were attracted by the possibility of higher wages and better living conditions; still others were forcibly resettled by Spanish officials and clerics attempting to consolidate the remnants of larger populations. In Honduras, for example, between 1582 and 1811, the number of native villages declined from 145 to 85.[93] Similar reductions or congregations of population occurred throughout Mexico, Central America, and the Andean region during the sixteenth century. In frontier areas such as northern Mexico and the Amazon Basin, clerics forced newly converted populations into mission settlements. While massive movements of population occurred throughout Spanish America, migration patterns differed from one region to another. Scholars estimate that in the Andean region, for example, between one-third and two-thirds of the region's indigenous inhabitants had relocated by the 1680s.[94] The migratory patterns that developed in Ecuador throughout the colonial era reveal the complexity and dynamic nature of these movements. The upheaval and violence of the Spanish conquest of the 1530s resulted in the flight of the native population away from Spanish-dominated centers of power in the highlands. By the end of the sixteenth century, however, this trend had reversed itself as many natives returned from the periphery to the center of the colonial system in search of improved wages and integration into the expanding colonial economy. Finally, as a result of the usurpation of the most productive native lands by colonists, during the late seventeenth and early eighteenth centuries, migration patterns altered once again, this time with movement away from the traditional centers of indigenous settlement in Quito and Otavalo into new regions to the south and east. As a result, by 1700, more than half of Ecuador's indigenous population lived somewhere other than their precontact ethnic homeland.[95]

While Spanish colonialism developed a series of complex institutions and practices to exploit indigenous labor, in the American colonies of Portugal, France, and England, the story was somewhat simpler, if no less devastating. Lacking densely settled native populations and easily exploited mineral resources, native labor was not the key to the success of these colonial enterprises. In Brazil, for example, the growth of a sugar plantation economy necessitated a steady supply of labor, but by the seventeenth century, the rapid decline of the region's indigenous population led to an increasing dependence on slaves imported from Africa.

As in Spanish America, migration of Brazil's native population occurred on a significant scale, with movement in two distinct directions: from the coast to the interior to escape the depredations of Portuguese settlers and slave raiders, and onto Jesuit missions. With regard to resettlement, the most sustained challenge to native communities came from the Jesuits, who began congregating natives into centrally located communities in the early 1550s. In many instances, natives resisted incorporation and ran away. A further deterrent to the success of the Jesuit missions was the hostility of many colonists, who regarded them as a challenge to their control of and access to native labor. By 1562, eleven missions hosted a total population of some thirty-four thousand natives.[96] But by the beginning of the seventeenth century, epidemics and slave raiding, even on the missions themselves, had taken their toll, and the number of natives in coastal Brazil had plummeted. During the next century, Portuguese colonists turned increasingly to the interior for native slaves.

In spite of the fact that French and English colonists failed to make extensive use of native labor, massive movements of indigenous populations also occurred in the areas controlled by these two nations. In these instances, migration was driven by rapidly increasing numbers of European immigrants, and as a result, the demand for productive agricultural lands accelerated throughout the eighteenth and nineteenth centuries. In many instances, this necessitated removing native residents from the land coveted by European settlers. In Virginia in the 1670s, the legislature passed a resolution stating that natives who left their villages without official permission forfeited their lands. In 1763, following the English defeat of the French at the end of the Seven Years War, the numbers of English colonists settling in Canada increased rapidly, and as a result, pressure on native lands throughout the region accelerated.

Just as the Spanish and Portuguese instituted policies designed to resettle or congregate native communities in the sixteenth and seventeenth centuries, the colonial governments of England and France, and later the United States and Canada, also established formal policies designed to relocate populations that stood in the way of European settlement. During the

1780s, for example, in order to facilitate the settlement of whites in Ohio, the government of the United States ordered the removal of the Miamis, Shawnees, and Delawares to the Great Lakes region. Between 1835 and 1838, the Cherokees of Georgia were forced west to the Mississippi on the infamous Trail of Tears, during which 10 to 20 percent of the population succumbed to disease, starvation, and exposure. Natives who refused to relocate were massacred by U.S. settlers.

The overall impact of forced, and to a lesser extent voluntary, migrations of indigenous peoples was to accelerate demographic decline and hinder recovery. Almost always, the land on which they resettled was less productive than the land they had left behind. Resettlement also facilitated the spread of infectious diseases, and when epidemics broke out, mortality rates were significantly higher than they would otherwise have been. In combination with the violence of war and slavery, migration and abusive labor systems also explain the failure of native American populations to recover as quickly or as completely as their counterparts in the Old World.

Conclusion

During the last twenty years, much of the blame for the demographic decline of native American populations has been placed almost exclusively on the introduction of smallpox, measles, bubonic plague, and other diseases from the Old World that triggered virgin soil epidemics of immense proportions. Certainly there is no denying the demographic devastation wrought by the waves of disease that repeatedly swept over the Americas after 1492, ultimately reducing most native populations by 75 percent or more. And while this study argues that all human populations react in similar ways to the same infectious organisms, nevertheless, in at least two respects, the situation that developed in the New World after 1492 with regard to disease and its demographic impact was unique. First, before the end of the fifteenth century, there is no evidence to suggest that any human population anywhere in the world ever experienced the nearly simultaneous arrival of three such highly virulent pathogens. The most devastating epidemics recorded in the Old World involved only one new pathogen at a time: the Plague of Athens, for example, was most likely precipitated by an outbreak of smallpox, while both the Plague of Justinian and the Black Death were caused by the appearance and spread of bubonic plague. Only in the Americas after 1492 and later in Oceania did human populations face wave upon wave of these previously unknown illnesses, often in conjunction with serious preexisting infections, within the span of several years.

Nevertheless, epidemic disease alone does not tell the whole story of this vast human tragedy. Any attempt to explain the prolonged demographic decline of indigenous American populations without carefully examining other factors would be incomplete and even misleading. Specifically, this book has argued that while epidemic disease accounts for much of that demographic decline, other factors specific to the phenomenon of European colonialism also played a significant role. Further, this study contends that it was European colonialism, in its various manifestations as practiced by the four European powers under consideration here, that differentiated the demographic experience of native American populations from that of populations in the Old World. The violence and social crises that resulted from the imposition of European colonialism greatly exacerbated native American mortality and ultimately undermined indigenous social, political, and economic institutions. Throughout the hemisphere, warfare accompanied initial contacts between Europeans and natives; famines followed in many areas as a result of the turmoil caused by epidemics and military conflicts. Slavery and other abusive labor practices as well as forced and voluntary migrations also took an enormous toll both in terms of native lives lost and sustained disruptions to local communities. In the long run, it was the disruption of day-to-day activities so crucial to the survival of any society that seriously undermined the demographic resilience of native American populations.

The examples of India and China, regions also colonized by Europeans, stand in marked contrast to the American experience. Because the indigenous peoples of these two regions had long been integrated into the unified disease pool of the Old World, virgin soil epidemics and severe demographic decline were not part of their colonial experience. Thus in both areas, native peoples were able to maintain their demographic dominance throughout the period of their colonization. In fact, Europeans had more reason to fear the disease environments of these two colonies than natives had to fear the introduction of diseases by Europeans. Because they were able to maintain their demographic advantage, the people of India and China were able to exert a greater degree of control over their fate at the hands of their colonizers than were native Americans, thus mitigating, at least to some extent, the impact of European colonialism. Undoubtedly similar situations involving virgin soil epidemics, catastrophic population decline, and delayed or failed demographic recovery occurred in various regions of the Old World before the modern era, although none would have assumed the scale and scope of the tragedy that played out in the New World. But as most of those incidents were never recorded or because the records have failed to survive, they have been lost to historians. One comparable situation that can be documented, however, is the case of Egypt in the wake of the bubonic plague epidemics of the fourteenth century. Following the deaths of as much as one-third of the population between 1347 and 1349, labor shortages and reduced agricultural production resulted in a series of famines, which, in turn, further reduced the population and drove frightened peasants into cities in search of food. Records reveal that in one region, the amount of land under cultivation forty years after the epidemics was only 4 percent of that under cultivation before 1347. Even more startling, however, is the fact that almost five centuries after the demographic catastrophe precipitated by the Black Death, the population of Egypt numbered only 3 million, whereas before 1347, that number has been estimated at approximately 8 million.[97] The failure of Egyptian authorities to respond to epidemic crises with effective public health measures, particularly quarantines, which proved so useful in reducing mortality rates in Europe, appears to explain this demographic anomaly. With the ascension of Muhammad Ali as viceroy of Egypt in 1805, the role of the Egyptian government in the area of public health changed dramatically, and over the next half century, the strict enforcement of quarantines, especially in port cities, significantly reduced and eventually eliminated outbreaks of bubonic plague. But in spite of the long-term decline and delayed recovery of the Egyptian population, today Egyptians constitute the majority within their homeland, and they remain active and influential participants in the political and economic life of their nation. This stands in marked contrast to the situation in the New World, where native Americans have never regained political or economic primacy in the territories they once controlled.

As with most things academic, there are actions and reactions—trends and countertrends. For almost five hundred years, Europe's stunning success at colonizing the Americas was attributed either to the skill and perspicacity of the colonizers or, alternately, to their violence and brutality. Twenty years ago, the pendulum began to swing the other way, and epidemic disease replaced violence as the primary explanation for the success of European colonialism and the decline of native populations. Now, at the beginning of the twenty-first century, a more complex view has emerged—one that acknowledges the devastating impact of virgin soil epidemics without minimizing the violence and destruction perpetrated by Europeans on New World populations. For too long, native Americans have been regarded as biologically and culturally exceptional, and as a result, they have been kept apart from the rest of humanity by scholars and the popular literature. This study attempts, in its own small way, to bring native Americans back into "the realm of planetary human experiences."[98]

Appendix • The Demographic Debate

*F*or [Indians] the arrival of Europeans marked the beginning of a long holocaust, although it came not in ovens, as it did for the Jews. The fires that consumed North American Indians were the fevers brought on by newly encountered diseases, the flashes of settlers' and soldiers' guns, the ravages of "firewater," the flames of villages and fields burned by the scorched-earth policy of vengeful Euro-Americans. The effects of this holocaust of North American Indians, like that of the Jews, was millions dead. In fact, the holocaust of the North American tribes was, in a way, even more destructive than that of the Jews, since many American Indian peoples became extinct.

Russell Thornton, *American Indian Holocaust and Survival*

To place this in a contemporary context, the ratio of native survivorship in the Americas following European contact was less than half of what the human survivorship ratio would be in the United States today if every single white person and every single black person died. The destruction of the Indians of the Americas was, far and away, the most massive act of genocide in the history of the world. That is why, as one historian aptly has said, far from the heroic and romantic heraldry that customarily is used to symbolize the European settlement of the Americas, the emblem most congruent with reality would be a pyramid of skulls.

David E. Stannard, *American Indian Holocaust*

Among other things, Columbus' journey was the first in a long process that eventually produced the United States of America, a daring experiment in democracy that in turn became a symbol and haven of individual liberty for people throughout the world. But the revolution that began with his voyages was far greater than that. It altered science, geography, philosophy, agriculture, law, religion, ethics, government—the sum, in other words, of what passed at the time as Western culture.

Robert Royal, *Columbus on Trial: 1492 v. 1992*

The Politics of Demography

As the preceding quotations illustrate, the Columbian Quincentenary of 1992 triggered a torrent of rhetoric concerning the long-term consequences of Columbus's arrival in the Americas. While the 500th anniversary of that momentous event has passed, the controversial issues it raised have not been forgotten, and proponents of both views continue to press their case. At one extreme are those who see Columbus and the Europeans who came after him as perpetrators of the largest genocide in human history, one that destroyed native American societies throughout the hemisphere. Critics of Columbus argued that rather than celebration, the anniversary of his arrival in the New World should be designated as a period of mourning, at the very least, a time to reflect on the magnitude of the tragedy that his actions initiated. At the other end of the political spectrum are those who view Columbus as hero and visionary and the changes that followed in the wake of his voyages as overwhelmingly positive. Columbus's supporters viewed the quincentenary as an occasion for eulogizing the man and for bringing to public attention the many benefits that we as Americans enjoy as a result of Columbus's bold actions.

For both sides this specific debate is only part of their larger political agendas: for critics to challenge many of the domestic and foreign policies of the governments of the United States and Canada, and for supporters to glorify the political and economic dominance of Western culture and, by extension, the U.S. government, at home and abroad at the end of the cold war. Clearly, events that took place over five hundred years ago continue to have an impact on life at the beginning of the new millennium. But regardless of political perspective, one cannot deny that following the arrival of Europeans in the Americas after 1492, a demographic decline of immense proportions began. And because the historical evidence is so overwhelming, one cannot deny that the introduction of Old World diseases played a major role in that decline.

The contentious nature of this debate has spilled over into the scholarly community, where historians, anthropologists, demographers, and others have staked out their own positions. Here, the most heated arguments have revolved around estimating the size of New World populations before 1492. The origins of this debate over the numbers of Amerindians inhabiting the hemisphere prior to contact with Europeans date from the years immediately following Columbus's arrival in the Americas. And scholarly debate has continued ever since, becoming increasingly heated, sometimes even acrimonious, especially during the second half of the twentieth century, and to date, the controversy shows no signs of abating. Why have normally dispassionate professionals invested so much time and energy on an issue for which there can never be a definitive answer? Why are these numbers so important? What difference does it make if the number of native Americans in 1492 was 8,000,000 or 200,000,000? The answer, according to one observer, is that

> our understanding of the European conquest—and with it the inception of global empire—is shaped by our sense of how badly indigenous populations were devastated during the first years of contact with Europeans. . . . The myth of European empire, wherein white colonists insert themselves into a sparsely inhabited land blessed with untapped resources, crumbles if the Americas had a large populace.[1]

The debate over the number of natives living in the Americas in 1492 revolves around three major issues: the level of social, political, and economic development attained by New World peoples before the arrival of Europeans; the degree to which European conquest and colonialism devastated Amerindian societies; and the nature and use of historical evidence. Were the Americas home to densely populated, highly developed societies, different from but equally as "civilized" as those of Europe? Or had the genetic and cultural isolation of New World populations hindered their demographic, economic, political, and technological development? Did the Spanish, Portuguese, British, and French wage wars of genocide against New World peoples in order to facilitate exploitation of the vast natural wealth of the Americas? How reliable is the historical evidence used by historians? What criteria do scholars employ when deciding whether or not to rely on a particular piece of information? And what about the use and alleged misuse of mathematical models and calculations by some demographic historians?

At least one historian has argued that since it is impossible to determine with any degree of accuracy what the size of the New World population was in 1492, it is better to abandon all attempts than to base an estimate on faulty logic and indirect evidence.[2] Others clearly believe it preferable to work with the data available, faulty though it may be, in order to posit what they consider to be reasonable estimates. What is at stake in this controversy is nothing less than an assessment of the level of development of native American societies as compared to those of the Old World, the exoneration or condemnation of European colonial powers for their role in the decline of New World populations, and the standards of argument and evidence that historians set for themselves.

Debate Over the Size of Native American Populations in 1492

The history of the study of native American demography is in itself instructive. Since the end of the fifteenth century, numerous individuals have offered population estimates for various regions of the Americas, but it was only during the twentieth century that sustained debate developed. Beginning in the 1920s, several scholars posited hemispheric population estimates of between 40,000,000 and 50,000,000, based on limited archaeological evidence and extensive extrapolation.[3] A decade later, an anthropologist and a historian significantly reduced these estimates to 8,000,000 and 13,000,000 respectively, arguing that they had not found sufficient evidence to support higher figures and that drastic demographic decline did not occur after 1492.[4] By the 1940s, others had undertaken regional studies, particularly of the Mesoamerican area, indicating the need for upward revision of these figures.[5] But it was not until the 1960s, when a large body of research had been accumulated, that the academic community began to take these higher projections seriously. Since that time, estimates of the precontact native population of the Americas have ranged from 33,300,000 to 145,000,000.[6] So, while the numbers have moved steadily upward since the 1930s, a wide disparity still exists, owing largely to differences in sources, methodologies, and assumptions.

On one side are those who insist that before 1500, the native population of the Americas numbered over 50,000,000 and that the islands of the Caribbean, Mesoamerica, and the Andean highlands, in particular, supported dense populations. In order to calculate estimates of native populations in specific regions, "high counters," as proponents of high estimates are often called by their critics, draw much of their evidence from early colonial documents, including censuses, tribute lists, descriptions of native settlements at the time of contact, and eyewitness accounts of military engagements during wars of conquest. In so doing, these researchers affirm the premise that sixteenth- and seventeenth-century Europeans could both count and estimate large numbers and that therefore these types of documentary evidence are generally reliable and of significant value to historians and other scholars. Two scholars noted for their use of early colonial documents in calculating the size of the precontact populations of Mexico and Hispaniola are physiologist Sherburne Cook and historian Woodrow Borah. In defending their use of an ecclesiastical account estimating that some 9,000,000 conversions and baptisms had taken place in Mexico between 1521 and 1536, they wrote, "Although later scholars have raised much objection to these numbers on the ground that they were exaggerations for personal glory, there is nothing inherently improbable in them, and they can be used as the basis for an estimate of the native population."[7] Cook and Borah had previously estimated the native population of central Mexico at 25,000,000 in 1518, a figure that prompted much heated debate.[8] In attempting to calculate the size of the indigenous population of Hispaniola in 1492, Cook and Borah began with the assumption that the estimates offered by Columbus and his contemporaries, many of which claimed over 1,000,000 inhabitants, were not only plausible, but actually underrepresented the size of the native population considerably. On the basis of these earliest figures, Cook and Borah plotted a population-time curve for the island, eventually arriving at a total population of 7,000,000 to 8,000,000 in 1492.[9]

In addition, proponents of high estimates argue that the introduction of European diseases and the brutality and exploitation of Spanish settlers significantly reduced demographic levels within a century following sustained contact with native societies. And in fact, high counters argue, in both the Andes and in large parts of North America, epidemics of Old World diseases arrived in advance of foreign conquerors and colonists, decimating native populations before Europeans ever laid eyes on them. If this was so, then scholars must also take into account the demographic impact of these earliest epidemics in order to estimate the size of some native populations.

If significant population decline did occur prior to the first Spanish censuses, then these sources do not accurately reflect the size of native communities. In such cases, researchers must do three things: first, they must try to determine what disease was most likely responsible for the outbreak; second, depending on the disease implicated in the epidemic, they must extrapolate a possible rate of mortality based on known death rates in epidemics of similar origin; and third, on the basis of this rate of mortality, they must correct the census figures, increasing the total to reflect the percentage loss, in order to arrive at an estimate of the population prior to the outbreak of the disease.

Thus in calculating the size of the precontact population of Peru, historian Noble David Cook first had to determine what diseases might have been responsible for two or three epidemics, one that occurred sometime between 1524 and 1526, a second that broke out in 1530 or 1531, and possibly a third that struck in 1531–1532. On the basis of limited evidence, Cook postulated that smallpox may have accounted for the first two outbreaks and measles for the third. He then calculated possible rates of mortality for the three epidemics, arriving at a range of 33 to 50 percent for the first and an additional 25 to 30 percent for the second and third epidemics that occurred before the arrival of the Pizarro expedition in 1532. On the basis of these calculations, Cook estimated that the indigenous population of Peru numbered between 3,000,000 and 8,000,000 in 1520.[10]

On the other side are those who argue that before 1492, the Americas were not as densely populated as the high counters have claimed, and that even in the highlands of Mexico and Peru, the number of inhabitants remained relatively low in comparison to the high estimates of their opponents. These scholars, often called "low counters," dismiss many contemporary Spanish sources as self-serving political documents, containing inflated figures. They also question the ability of sixteenth-century Europeans to provide reliable estimates of the populations with which they came into contact. One critic of high estimates, historian David Henige, argued that sixteenth-century Spaniards "had trouble counting each other," so how, he wondered, could they possibly be relied upon to offer accurate estimates of groups of people with whom they often came into contact only briefly and often under the chaotic conditions of war?[11] For example, Hernán Cortés, conqueror of Mexico, claimed that in 1520, Spanish forces encountered Aztec armies numbering up to 150,000. Low counters argue that Cortés's desire to enhance his reputation as a military leader and curry favor with the king of Spain motivated him to inflate the ranks of the Aztec armies, rendering this figure completely unreliable.[12]

Furthermore, advocates of low estimates argue that although native populations certainly declined after the arrival of Europeans, the drop was far less dramatic than the high counters claim. According to the low counters, given the relatively small size of the Amerindian population at contact, the impact of epidemic diseases was also less devastating than their opponents have argued. Supporters of this thesis argue that censuses conducted by Spanish officials during the first century after the arrival of Europeans accurately represent the size of the precontact population. A census of the native population of highland Ecuador, made some twenty years after the Spanish conquest of the region, provides a useful illustration. In 1561, a Spanish official, Juan Matienzo de Peralta, issued a report, based on a census taken two years earlier, stating that some 270,000 natives resided within his jurisdiction. In spite of the many documents attesting to widespread violence and disease in the years between 1534 and 1559, low counters regard this figure as a more or less accurate representation of the number of native inhabitants in highland Ecuador before the arrival of Europeans. Clearly, this approach has the effect of reducing the size of the precontact population and minimizing the impact of Old World diseases.

High counters, on the other hand, argue that in addition to the many thousands who lost their lives as a result of military engagements between natives and Spaniards, several major epidemics swept through the area between 1520 and 1559, drastically reducing the size of the precontact population. Therefore, they argue, this figure underrepresents the size of Ecuador's Amerindian population significantly. Several scholars who argue that Matienzo de Peralta's figure is too low have calculated totals ranging from 838,600 to 1,080,000.[13]

North America is another area where low counters argue that Old World diseases arrived only following sustained contact with colonists, not during long periods of short-term and temporary contacts, and that the number and extent of epidemics during the colonial period were far more limited than their opponents claim. In disputing the claims that epidemic disease preceded Europeans in many areas of the Americas, significantly reducing native populations, Henige charged, "that they have been unable to demonstrate this even once is certainly not inconsequential, but, more seriously yet, they cannot disprove its polar opposite—that in *no* case did this occur. The claim, then, is epistemologically vacuous, existing merely of and for itself, with ideological status only. For the highcounters, this is enough."[14]

Methods of Estimating Precontact Native Populations

In their attempts to calculate the size of the Amerindian population before contact, both high counters and low counters have adopted a variety of methods, and some of these techniques have generated as much controversy as the numbers themselves. One of the earliest and most widely used of all methods is the guesstimate: lacking specific demographic information, some scholars have made informed guesses, based on their impressions of the size of a particular population. This appears to be the way the seventeenth-century Jesuit Giovanni Battista Riccioli arrived at his hemispheric estimate of 200,000,000, for he offers no clue as to how he obtained this figure.[15] Some have simply borrowed the figures of other researchers, then adjusted them to suit their own needs. For example, linguist Angel Rosenblat adopted anthropologist Julian

Steward's estimate of the native population of Central America (736,000) and adjusted it upward by 64,000 without explanation.[16]

Another popular method involves the creation of analogies between known and unknown populations. Anthropologist Alfred Kroeber, a low counter, calculated the native population of North America using individual tribal estimates; he then based his estimate for the population of South America "on the assumption that the relation of Peru to the remainder of South America was similar to the relation of Mexico to the remainder of North America."[17] Obviously such a sweeping assumption may not be warranted because it fails to take into account important environmental and cultural differences between the two regions.

Another method involves the use of population densities. Having calculated the number of persons who resided within a particular area, some have applied that same density to a wider region of unknown population. Anthropologist Henry Dobyns employed this method in arriving at his estimate of 18,000,000 natives in North America, the highest to date.[18] But again, environmental and cultural distinctions between regions and societies render such comparisons invalid.

Especially for high counters, the introduction of epidemic diseases from the Old World to the New played an important role in shaping demographic patterns. As a result, some scholars have used a method called epidemic correction to ascertain the size of particular populations that may have experienced significant diminution either before the arrival of Europeans or before reliable censuses were taken. For example, in analyzing various methods of estimating the precontact population of Peru, historian Noble David Cook calculated mortality rates associated with six epidemics that occurred between 1524 and 1615. Subsequently he used these figures to project back, arriving at an estimated population of 3,750,000 to 8,000,000 in 1520.[19] A major problem with this method is that the documentary and archaeological evidence is insufficient to allow reliable calculation of mortality.

Using a method known as backward projection, some have extrapolated back from known rates of decline in order to establish the size of earlier populations. Thus mathematician Rudolph Zambardino arrived at his estimate of 5,130,000 for the precontact population of the Andes by calculating the rate of decline from 1570 to 1600 and projecting it back to 1520.[20] Others have devised depopulation ratios, based on the ratio between a known population in 1492 and its nadir, or low point; these ratios are then applied to wider areas, sometimes even the hemisphere as a whole. Dobyns did just that when he calculated "standard" hemispheric depopulation ratios of 20 to 1 and 25 to 1, yielding a total population of 90,043,000 to 112,533,750 in 1492.[21] Once again, the major criticism of this method is that applying a depopulation ratio from one community to societies in vastly different circumstances yields results with an unacceptably wide margin of error.

Others have adopted an ecological approach, estimating population based on the carrying capacity of the land. This method is based on the Malthusian assumption that populations will expand to the limits of their available food supply. Thus by calculating the amount of land available for agricultural production and the amount of food produced per hectare, historian Noble David Cook estimated that as many as 13,000,000 persons could have lived in Peru before 1520.[22] The problem with this method is that its underlying assumption may be false because not every society expands to the limits of its available resources.

The techniques of demographic archaeologists and paleopathologists have also been brought to bear on the debate, and in many cases, the archaeological evidence suggests severe population decline either shortly before or immediately after contact with Europeans.[23] Changing settlement patterns among native inhabitants in the lower Mississippi Valley during the sixteenth century, for example, indicate that population loss coincided with the arrival of the de Soto expedition in 1541. Thus by the time sustained contact developed with Europeans during the late seventeenth century, the number of Amerindians in the lower Mississippi Valley already had declined precipitously.[24]

Finally, in an attempt to bring some scientific rationale to the issue, some have turned to mathematics and, most recently, computer simulations. Zambardino used logarithmic scales and extrapolation to arrive at a precontact population of 1,000,000 on the island of Hispaniola, and historian Thomas Whitmore devised "a system dynamics computer simulation" to analyze postcontact population decline in the Basin of Mexico.[25]

But it is the implications of these calculations even more than the numbers themselves that continue to generate controversy. High counters argue that population density is directly related to the degree of technological and cultural advancement of a society. Hence to accept the premise that Mesoamerica and the central Andes were densely populated in 1492, one must also accept that the societies of these regions were not only not primitive but had achieved levels of political and economic development equal to or greater than those of Europe and so could sustain such large numbers of people. If in fact something approaching 100,000,000 natives resided in the Americas in 1492, they outnumbered the populations of Europe and Russia combined, estimates of which range from 70,000,000 to 88,000,000. Linguists have also proposed that the level of cultural diversity was probably greater in the New World than in the Old, based in part on the large number of languages spoken by native Americans.[26] And if one does accept the arguments and numbers of the high counters, it then follows that a demographic tragedy of immense proportions began in the Americas at the end of the fifteenth century. But low counters argue that the ambiguous evidence and faulty methodologies of many high counters render their conclusions worthless.

While this debate centers on events that happened centuries ago, it also has immediate, practical relevance. Many native Americans argue that acceptance of low precontact population estimates supports the notion of the Americas, especially North America, as wilderness and its inhabitants as savages. This view of North America as a nearly vacant landscape allowed European governments, and later the governments of the United States and Canada, to justify seizure of native lands.[27]

Given the nature of this difficult and emotional issue, and because the existing evidence lends itself to such varying interpretations, it may never be possible for high and low counters to resolve their differences. And while some scholars have assumed a middle ground, debate is certain to continue for many years.

The Numbers

In light of this controversy, what was the size of the native American population in 1492, and how have scholars gone about determining that figure? Let us begin with a review of the data for each area, starting in North America, bearing in mind that not all regions have received equal scholarly attention and that in fact some areas have received little or none. Historians, demographers, archaeologists, and others have conducted more research on native populations in North America, Mesoamerica, and the Andes than in other locations, in the first case because of the availability of financial resources and in the latter two cases because more physical and documentary evidence remains. Conversely, we still know relatively little about native populations in more remote areas such as the Arctic and southern South America.

North America

Estimates of the native population of North America at the end of the fifteenth century range from a high of 18,000,000 to a low of 900,000. The larger figure, that offered by Dobyns in 1983, is based on the Malthusian theory that human populations tend to increase to the maximum that their natural resources will allow. Dividing native North American societies into agricultural and nonagricultural, Dobyns used censuses, estimates of historic settlement sizes, depopulation ratios, and carrying capacities to calculate population densities for large areas of North America. On the basis of these figures (persons per square kilometer), he posited a population of some 14,000,000 people living in agricultural communities. In addition, Dobyns calculated that some 4,500,000 nonhorticulturalists also occupied territory in various areas of North America, bringing the total North American Indian population to more than 18,000,000.[28]

Dobyns's high estimate has been roundly criticized by many low counters. Using data drawn from studies of specific localities, Dobyns applied these figures to huge areas, assuming the same population density throughout. Such assumptions are not justified by the evidence, and furthermore, this method does not allow for the regional variations that surely existed. In other instances, he offers no clue as to the basis for his calculations, as in the case of the greater Mississippi River Valley, where he writes, "Horticultural peoples estimated to include 5,250,000 individuals lived there, averaging 2.53 persons per km²."[29] No citation follows. All of these calculations are highly speculative, yet Dobyns writes with a certainty that does not adequately address problems with the evidence or the tentative nature of his conclusions.

Kroeber's figure of 900,000 for North America, published in 1934, was derived from his adjustments to an earlier estimate of 1,150,000 by ethnographer James Mooney.[30] Mooney compiled figures on tribal populations, some of which were based on censuses, others on observations of European colonists, and still others on documents compiled as late as the mid-nineteenth century. Mooney's estimates, therefore, were often incomplete and would not reflect population decline if such had occurred before sustained contact with European settlers. Furthermore, careful review of Mooney's research reveals that his figures were intended as low estimates; thus Kroeber's reduction of them was unjustified.[31]

Many scholars have criticized both Dobyns's high figure and Kroeber's low one on the basis of methodologies as well as conclusions. As a result, others have offered their own estimates of the size of the native population of North America at the end of the fifteenth century. In 1976, anthropologist Douglas Ubelaker, a supporter of low estimates, noted that "historically, estimates have shifted from conservative in 1910 to liberal in the '20s, back to conservative in the '30s and '40s and then to liberal again in the '60s."[32] Almost twenty years later, we might add that most estimates remained high through the 1960s and 1970s, with increasing support for lower numbers during the 1980s and 1990s. Nevertheless, many scholars continue to accept moderate to high estimates. In general, this historical pattern also holds true for estimates of native populations throughout the hemisphere.

Years before the publication of Kroeber's estimate in 1939, geographer Karl Sapper and ethnologist William Christie MacLeod offered totals of

2,500,000 to 3,500,000 and 3,000,000, respectively, for North America, based on calculations of carrying capacity and population density.[33] But these higher figures were largely ignored in favor of Kroeber's low estimate, which enjoyed wide acceptance until the 1960s. Then in 1966 Dobyns dismissed previous figures as absurdly low, arguing for a North American population of some 9,000,000 to 12,000,000, based on the calculation of

Table A.1 Estimates of the Native Population of North America at Contact			
Date	Source	Estimate	Methodology
1924	Sapper	2.5–3,500,000	carrying capacity
1928	Mooney	1,152,950	tribal estimates
1928	MacLeod	3,000,000	carrying capacity and population density
1934	Kroeber	900,000	adjusted Mooney
1949	Steward	1,000,000	based on Kroeber and Rosenblat (1949)
1954	Rosenblat	1,000,000	adjusted Kroeber
1966	Dobyns	9.8–12,250,000	depopulation ratio/20:1 and 25:1
1969	Driver	3,500,000	depopulation ratio/10:1
1976	Ubelaker	2,171,125	revised Mooney's tribal estimates
1976	Denevan	4,400,000	doubled Ubelaker—epidemic correction
1983	Dobyns	18,000,000	carrying capacity and population density
1983	Hughes	5–10,000,000	carrying capacity
1987	Ramenofsky	12,000,000	demographic archaeology and depopulation ratio
1987	Thornton	7,000,000	mean of Dobyns's depopulation ratio
1988	Ubelaker	1,894,350	revised tribal estimates
1990	Sale	15,000,000	guess
1992	Jaffee	1,250,000	guess
1992	Stiffarm	15,000,000	based on Sale
1992	Stannard	8–12,000,000	review of literature
1992	Denevan	3,800,000	revision—doubled Ubelaker

regional nadirs at the end of the nineteenth century multiplied by depopulation ratios of 20 to 1 and 25 to 1.[34] Dobyns's first estimate generated much heated controversy and spurred many scholars to undertake their own research on the demographics of precontact America.

Among those who responded to Dobyns's challenge was anthropologist Harold Driver. In 1969, Driver calculated that the Indian population of the continental United States had reached its nadir of 250,000 in 1890. Recognizing that some significant degree of demographic decline had occurred, he multiplied the nadir figure by a factor of 10 in order to arrive at a precontact native population of 2,500,000. Using similar methods, Driver also calculated that the aboriginal populations of Canada, Greenland, and Alaska probably numbered approximately 1,000,000, bringing his total for North America to 3,500,000.[35]

On the basis of tribe-by-tribe estimates submitted for the Smithsonian Institution's revision of the *Handbook of North American Indians* in 1976, Ubelaker calculated that the native population of North America numbered 2,171,125 around 1500. He based this figure on new and revised estimates of tribal areas that compared directly to those used by Mooney and Kroeber. According to Ubelaker, this 88 percent increase over Kroeber's total of 900,000 was due not only to new sources and methods, but also to a willingness on the part of scholars to accept increasingly large population estimates.[36] Later in 1976, geographer William Denevan published his estimate of 4,400,000, based on a doubling of Ubelaker's figure, which he argued was too low and failed to take into account the massive depopulation that occurred during the first century after contact.[37]

Debate continued during the 1980s with the publication of several more estimates. Historian J. Donald Hughes offered an estimate of from 5,000,000 to 10,000,000, based on his calculations of carrying capacity.[38] In 1987, sociologist Russell Thornton estimated a precontact native population of some 7,000,000, 5,000,000 in the continental United States and 2,000,000 more in Canada. Thornton arrived at these figures by applying the mean of Dobyns's depopulation ratio to Driver's nadir population of 250,000 at the end of the nineteenth century.[39] On the basis of archaeological research at three test sites that revealed high levels of depopulation after contact, Ann F. Ramenofsky calculated a precontact population of some 12,000,000.[40]

More recently, both Ubelaker and Denevan have revised their calculations. Based on further revisions of specific tribal populations submitted for the *Handbook of North American Indians* in 1988, Ubelaker lowered his estimate from some 2,200,000 to 1,894,350.[41] Subsequently, in 1992, Denevan adjusted his estimate from 4,400,000 to 3,800,000, again based on a doubling of Ubelaker's totals, which he argued failed to correct for demographic decline in the decades immediately following contact.[42]

What can one conclude from the previous discussion? First, that no agreement exists as to the size of the native population of North America at the end of the fifteenth century. Second, that since we will probably never know how many individuals lived in North America before contact, the best that we can do is to arrive at a range of population that appears reasonable in light of the evidence available to us. Given Ubelaker's careful assessment of tribal estimates (1,894,350) and the growing body of archaeological evidence indicating severe depopulation during the sixteenth and seventeenth centuries, Denevan's doubling of Ubelaker's total does not appear unjustified.

Mexico

When the Spanish arrived in central Mexico in 1519, they encountered dense native populations, organized into highly structured political and economic units. The first Europeans to visit the Mexica capital recorded their wonder and amazement at what they saw:

> With such wonderful sights to gaze on we did not know what to say, or if this was real that we saw before our eyes. On the land side there were great cities, and on the lake many more. The lake was crowded with canoes. At intervals along the causeway there were many bridges, and before us was the great city of Mexico.[43]

> The great city [of Tenochtitlán] is as big as Seville or Cordoba. There is also one square twice as big as that of Salamanca, with arcades all around, where more than sixty thousand people come each day to buy and sell, and where every kind of merchandise produced in these lands is found.[44]

Estimates of the size of the native population of Mexico on the eve of the Spanish conquest range from 3,200,000 to 58,178,000. The enormity of the disparity between these two figures is indicative of the intensity of the controversy among scholars. In fact, debate over the size of Mexico's native population began even before the fall of the Aztec capital in 1521, when Cortés's estimates of native armies numbering as many as 150,000 generated skeptical debate at the Spanish court, just as they continue to do today.

But more was at stake than just Cortés's reputation as a brilliant military commander: ascertaining the number of natives living in Mexico at the time of the Spanish conquest had important economic significance.

Table A.2 Estimates of the Native Population of Mexico at Contact			
Date	Source	Estimate	Methodology
1924	Sapper	12–15,000,000	carrying capacity
1934	Kroeber	3,200,000	"impressions" and comparisons to North America
1949	Steward	4,500,000	adjusted Kroeber
1954	Rosenblat	4,500,000	review of literature
1963	Cook and Borah	25,200,000	colonial documents and depopulation ratios
1966	Dobyns	30–37,500,000	depopulation ratios/20:1 and 25:1
1969	Driver	20,000,000	reduction of Dobyns
1970	Sanders	11,400,000	archaeological, ecological, and documentary evidence
1976	Denevan	21,400,000	average of Cook and Borah and Sanders plus totals for outside areas
1978	Slicher von Bath	21,400,000	adjusted Cook and Borah
1981	Zambardino	8–10,000,000	extrapolation to 1518 from postcolonial estimates
1988	Dobyns	58,178,666	guess
1991	Whitmore	16,000,000	computer simulation
1992	Denevan	17,200,000	average of Zambardino, Sanders, Slicher van Bath, and Whitmore

In order to distribute encomiendas to his leading military commanders and supporters, Cortés needed to determine the size and location of native settlements. Thus some of the earliest sources of demographic data for Mexico are censuses related to the granting of encomiendas. In addition, the Mexica government also kept written records, some of which contain valuable information concerning their system of taxation, including the types and amounts of tribute collected.

Officials of the Catholic Church, eager to demonstrate their diligence and success to their superiors in Madrid and Rome, also kept records of the number of Amerindians converted to Christianity. In some cases, priests claimed to have baptized thousands of natives a day, leading some to question not only the depth and sincerity of the conversions, but the veracity of the figures. Just as Cortés's descriptions of enormous native armies were suspect, so too were many of these conversion figures. Nevertheless, modern scholars have relied on both sets of data in their attempts to calculate the size of Mexico's precontact population.

While much of this demographic data proved highly controversial during the early colonial period, by the beginning of the twentieth century it had been discredited or forgotten. Kroeber did not employ any of these sources when, in 1934, he placed the number of Indians living in "High-culture Mexico," which included Guatemala and El Salvador, at 3,200,000. Rather, he based his calculations on "impressions" and comparisons with population densities north of the Rio Grande.[45] He also dismissed Sapper's totals of 12,000,000 to 15,000,000 as highly inflated.[46] Kroeber's low count enjoyed wide acceptance during the next two decades, and the estimates of Steward and Rosenblat, both of whom placed the precontact population of Mexico at 4,500,000, adjusted Kroeber's figure upward only slightly.[47]

In 1963, Cook and Borah revolutionized the study of pre-Columbian demography, not only for Mexico but for all of the Americas, with the publication of their estimate of 25,200,000 for central Mexico.[48] In this and subsequent publications, Cook and Borah utilized precisely those sources so long neglected by other scholars, namely the earliest Spanish and native documents, including conquerors' reports, church records, and tribute lists, both Mexica and Spanish. The work of these two authors received widespread attention, attracting many supporters and detractors. While some criticized the problematic sources, assumptions, and calculations on which this work rested, since 1963, higher estimates have been met with greater acceptance. Three years later, Dobyns offered an even higher figure of 30,000,000 to 37,500,000, based on nadir populations and a depopulation ratio of 20 to 1.[49] He would later revise that figure upward to some 58,000,000, the highest estimate for Mexico by far.[50]

Others argued for totals somewhat closer to Cook and Borah's own: Driver—20,000,000; Denevan—21,400,000; and Slicher von Bath—21,400,000.[51] Utilizing archaeological, ecological, and documentary evidence, archaeologist William Sanders calculated that the population of the Basin of Mexico numbered approximately 2,900,000 in 1519.[52]

Compared to Cook and Borah's totals for this same region, this represented a reduction of more than half. Extrapolation from this ratio to Cook and Borah's total for all of central Mexico yielded a population of 11,400,000 in 1519.[53] Zambardino was also highly critical of Cook and Borah's methods and proposed his own estimate of 8,000,000 to 10,000,000.[54] Most recently, geographer Thomas Whitmore employed computer simulation to reconstruct the precontact population of central Mexico, arriving at a figure of 16,000,000.[55] Denevan, too, reduced his total for Mexico by 4,200,000 to 17,200,000.[56]

What, then, appears to be the most reasonable estimate of Mexico's native population on the eve of the Spanish conquest? Certainly the archaeological and documentary evidence does not support either the highest figure, 58,177,666, or the lowest figure, 3,200,000. The methodology employed by Whitmore in his computer simulation has received wide praise, and his estimate of 16,000,000 appears reasonable, if still a bit low. Denevan's total of 17,200,000, based on the average of Zambardino's, Sander's, Slicher von Bath's, and Whitmore's calculations, may thus represent the most accurate to date. Therefore a population of from 16,000,000 to 18,000,000 appears well within the range of possibility.

Central America

Following the military conquest of Tenochtitlán in 1521, the Spanish turned their attention to the native societies of Central America. In southern Mexico, Guatemala, El Salvador, and Belize, they encountered densely populated Maya city-states. Farther south in Honduras, Nicaragua, Costa Rica, and Panama, chiefdoms dominated large agricultural populations. The Spanish met fierce resistance in many parts of Central America; nevertheless, by the 1530s much of the isthmus had been brought under European control. As in the case of Mexico, the conquerors of Central America also distributed encomiendas to their followers; thus gathering information on the size of native populations was crucial during the early colonial period and these documents constitute many of the most valuable sources of modern demographers.

In reviewing estimates of the size of the native population of Central America at contact, one major problem emerges: some scholars have calculated the population for only one particular area, not for the region as a whole. Therefore we will limit our discussion to only those figures that cover the entire Central American area.

Estimates of the size of the precontact population of Central America range from a low of 800,000, offered by Rosenblat in 1954, to Dobyns's high of 13,500,000. Rosenblat based his figure in part on the calculations of Kroeber, who posited a total of 3,300,000 for Mexico and Central

America combined.[57] Once again, Dobyns offered the highest estimate, 13,500,000, which he arrived at by applying his depopulation ratio of 20 to 1 to the nadir population of the region.[58]

One of the earliest estimates for Central America was offered by Sapper in 1924. Based on theories of carrying capacity, he calculated the precontact population at 5,000,000 to 6,000,000.[59] In 1949, Steward proposed a total of 736,000, exclusive of Guatemala.[60] Driver halved Dobyns's figure in order to arrive at his own estimate of 6,000,000.[61] Using a variety of sources, including population data for specific regions such as Panama (1,000,000), Nicaragua (1,000,000), and El Salvador (500,000) and comparative estimates for Honduras and Belize (750,000), Costa Rica (400,000), and Guatemala (2,000,000), in 1976, Denevan calculated 5,650,000 for the region as a whole.[62] Historian William Sherman, on the other hand, posited a total of 2,250,000, based on Rosenblat's review of the demographic literature.[63] In 1992, Denevan revised his figures in light of new research on the region, arriving at a new estimate of 5,625,000.[64] Most recently, historical geographer W. George Lovell and historian Christopher Lutz calculated a total of 5,105,000, based on their own studies of Guatemala and the recent research of others.[65] Interestingly, the recent estimates of Denevan and Lovell and Lutz closely approximate the estimate proposed by Sapper in 1924. I also find Sapper's range of 5,000,000 to 6,000,000 most reasonable, and I adopt it here for the purposes of this study.

Table A.3 Estimates of the Native Population of Central America at Contact			
Date	Source	Estimate	Methodology
1924	Sapper	5–6,000,000	carrying capacity
1949	Steward	736,000[*]	population density
1954	Rosenblat	800,000	adjusted Steward
1966	Dobyns	10.8–13,500,000	depopulation ratio/ 20:1 and 25:1
1969	Driver	6,000,000	half of Dobyns
1976	Denevan	5,650,000	review of literature and comparisons
1979	Sherman	2,250,000	review of literature
1992	Denevan	5,625,000	review of literature
1995	Lovell and Lutz	5,105,000	review of literature

[*]Excludes Guatemala.

The Caribbean

A review of the demographic literature on the precontact population of the Caribbean reveals that one island, Hispaniola, has attracted more attention than any other. Hispaniola, the island that today encompasses the nations of Haiti and the Dominican Republic, became the focus of Spanish conquest and settlement following the first Columbus expedition in 1492. It was here that the institution of encomienda was first introduced to the Americas, and it was here that the disastrous decline of native populations began. A number of observers commented on the rapid decline of the native population, which had almost completely disappeared fifty years after contact, and they compared the almost extinct population to the large number of Amerindians inhabiting the island when Columbus arrived in 1492. These contemporary accounts have provided modern scholars with information on which to base their own calculations. Thus when studying the Caribbean, one must deal with two sets of figures: those for Hispaniola and those for the region as a whole.

Estimates of the size of the native population of Hispaniola in 1492 range from a low of 60,000 to a high of 8,000,000. The low figure, offered by historian Charles Verlinden, was based on simple backward projection from two censuses conducted in 1514 and 1508.[66] Cook and Borah arrived at the higher estimate by using contemporary accounts to arrive at a figure of 3,770,000 for 1496, developing a population curve and projecting back from that date.[67] But their methodology has been widely criticized; one scholar described it as "a towering edifice constructed entirely of non-load bearing 'possible to probable' assumptions."[68]

Las Casas, encomendero, priest, and defender of native Americans, claimed that some 3,000,000 to 4,000,000 natives inhabited the island in 1492.[69] But he contradicted himself, writing elsewhere that the island's population numbered only 1,000,000 when Columbus arrived.[70] Several other sixteenth-century writers also agreed with the 1,000,000 figure.[71] At least one, Nicolas Federman, a German immigrant, disagreed, recording the number as 500,000.[72]

Arguing that contemporary estimates were grossly inflated, Rosenblat calculated a total of 100,000.[73] Historian Frank Moya Pons first arrived at a figure of 600,000 but later decreased his estimate to 377,559, based on his projected population for 1503 and the rate of decline to 1492.[74] On the basis of contemporary accounts and logarithmic scale, Zambardino accepted an estimate of some 1,000,000.[75] Denevan reduced his initial estimate of 1,950,000, based on the average of Cook and Borah's 8,000,000 and Rosenblat's 100,000, to 1,000,000, following the publication of Zambardino's figure.[76]

Most recently, historian Noble David Cook entered the fray, offering

Table A.4 Estimates of the Native Population of Hispaniola at Contact			
Date	Source	Estimate	Methodology
1517	Las Casas	3–4,000,000	guess
1518	de Zuazo	1,130,000	based on Columbus's census
1529–1530	Federman	500,000	not clear
1954	Rosenblat	100,000	review of literature
1971	Cook and Borah	8,000,000	logarithmic projection and population curve
1973	Verlinden	60,000	backward projection from 1514 and 1508 censuses
1976	Denevan	1,950,000	average of Cook and Borah and Rosenblat
1978	Zambardino	1,000,000	review of literature and logarithmic scale
1987	Moya Pons	377,559	increased1508 census by one-third
1992	Denevan	1,000,000	based on Zambardino
1993	N. D. Cook	500–750,000	based on Federman and corrected Moya Pons

an estimate of from 500,000 to 750,000, based on the 1529 figure of Federman and an adjusted calculation of Moya Pons's 377,559. But he also conceded that "the Alonso de Zuazo–Pedro Martir de Angleria figures of 1,130,000–1,200,000 may provide a conservative upper limit for estimates."[77] For our purposes, therefore, a range of from 500,000 to 1,000,000 appears reasonable.

Considerably less attention has been focused on the Caribbean as a whole, but several scholars have offered estimates, ranging from 200,000 to 5,850,000. Kroeber's low figure was not based on any empirical data, while Denevan calculated his total of almost 6,000,000 by combining his estimate for the population of Hispaniola (1,950,000) and 3,900,000 for the other islands, based on Rosenblat's claim that the inhabitants of these islands numbered twice as many as those of Hispaniola.[78] Steward and Rosenblat both supported low figures for the region, 220,000 and 300,000 respectively.[79] In his 1966 article, Dobyns postulated a total of 443,000 to 553,750 for the region as a whole, based on backward projection from a nadir population of 22,150 in 1570.[80] A higher estimate of 2,000,000 to 3,500,000 was offered by Sapper in 1924.[81] This figure agrees closely with Denevan's revised total of 3,000,000 published in 1992, based on a population of 1,000,000 on Hispaniola and double that for the rest of the region.[82] Having already accepted an estimate of 500,000 to 1,000,000 natives on the island of Hispaniola alone, the figures of Kroeber, Steward, and Rosenblat are clearly too low. Denevan himself reduced his earlier estimate of 5,850,000 to 3,000,000. Thus Sapper and Denevan's estimates of 2,000,000 to 3,000,000 appear most reasonable.

The Andes

Estimates of the size of the native population of the Andes at contact range from a low of 2,000,000 to 3,000,000 to a high of 30,000,000 to 37,000,000. Among the low counters are Kroeber, Rowe, Steward, and Rosenblat, all of whose methodologies we have discussed previously; they are joined by Zambardino and archaeologist Daniel Shea.[83] Shea calculated the rate of decline in the central Andes between 1581 and 1613 and projected it back

Date	Source	Estimate	Methodology
Table A.5 Estimates of the Native Population of the Caribbean at Contact			
1924	Sapper	2–3,500,000	carrying capacity
1934	Kroeber	200,000	analogy with Mexico and North America
1949	Steward	225,000	adjusted Kroeber
1954	Rosenblat	300,000	review of literature
1966	Dobyns	443,000–553,750	depopulation ratio/20:1 and 25:1
1976	Denevan	5,850,000	average of Cook and Borah and Rosenblat for Hispaniola and double that for rest of area
1992	Denevan	3,000,000	based on Zambardino's 1,000,000 for Hispaniola and double that for rest of area

to obtain a population of some 2,000,000 to 3,000,000 in 1520. Zambardino, who also dealt only with the central Andean region, arrived at his estimate of 5,130,000 by figuring the rate of decline from 1570 to 1600 and projecting it back. Both Shea and Zambardino dealt only with the central Andes, and they did not take into account the fact that mortality rates may have been higher in the period before 1570; thus their calculations minimize the number of pre-Columbian inhabitants.

Table A.6 Estimates of the Native Population of the Andes at Contact			
Date	Source	Estimate	Methodology
1924	Sapper	12–15,000,000	carrying capacity
1934	Kroeber	3,000,000	analogy with Mexico and North America
1946	Rowe	6,000,000	depopulation ratios: sierra 4:1/coast 16:1 and 25:1
1949	Steward	6,130,000	population density
1954	Rosenblat	4,750,000	adjusted Steward estimate
1966	Dobyns	30–37,000,000	depopulation ratios/20:1 and 25:1
1970	Smith	12,100,000	depopulation ratios: sierra 3:1/coast 58:1
1976	Shea	2–3,000,000	backward projection, rate of decline, 1581–1613
1976	Denevan	11,500,000	average of Smith and Shea
1977	Wachtel	11,200,000	depopulation ratio 4:1
1981	Cook	13,000,000	carrying capacity
1981	Zambardino	5,130,000	backward projection, rate of decline 1570–1600
1992	Denevan	15,700,000	average of adjusted totals of Cook, Wachtel, and Smith
1992	Verano	6–13,000,000	review of literature

Among the high counters are Sapper and Dobyns, whose methods we have already reviewed, as well as Smith, Denevan, Wachtel, and Cook.[84] Geographer C. T. Smith worked with two sixteenth-century censuses of the tributary population of the central Andes, calculating an overall ratio of nine individuals to every one tributary (tributaries to total population). He then employed depopulation ratios of 3 to 1 for the sierra (three out of every four people died) and 58 to 1 for coastal areas (fifty-eight out of every fifty-nine people died) in order to obtain a total of 12,100,000. Denevan arrived at his estimate of 11,500,000 by averaging the figures of Smith and Shea, also taking into account the Andean populations of Colombia and Venezuela. French historian Nathan Wachtel applied a depopulation ratio of 4 to 1, producing a total of 11,200,000. Historian Noble David Cook utilized a variety of methods in his study of the native population of Peru. His conclusion, based on the backward projection of regional rates of decline, posits some 9,000,000 natives in Peru alone in 1520; using calculations of carrying capacity, he offers an estimate of 13,000,000 for the entire Andean region. In 1992, Denevan revised his earlier estimate; based on the average of adjusted totals from Cook, Wachtel, and Smith, his total of 15,700,000 showed a substantial increase over his figure for 1976. Having reviewed the literature, anthropologist John Verano offered a range encompassing both low and high estimates, 6,000,000 to 13,000,000.[85] My own review of the evidence indicates that a population in the range of 13,000,000 to 15,000,000 appears reasonable.

Lowland South America

The native peoples of lowland South America inhabited ecologically and climatically diverse expanses of Amazonia, southern Brazil, Argentina, central Chile, Uruguay, eastern Colombia, Venezuela, and the Guianas. In comparison to the native inhabitants of North America, Mexico, and the Andes, the Amerindian populations of these vast regions have received far less scholarly attention, and the studies that have been conducted often focused on specific areas and not the entire lowland region. Nevertheless, a number of scholars have attempted to estimate the precontact population, producing figures ranging from a low of 1,000,000 to a high of 9,000,000 to 11,250,000. Arguing that lowland South America's native societies were analogous in many respects to the hunter-gatherer societies of North America, Kroeber offered a total of 1,000,000, while Dobyns's depopulation ratios of 20 to 1 and 25 to 1 produced a range of from 9,000,000 to 11,250,000.[86] Sapper based his estimate of from 3,000,000 to 5,000,000 on carrying capacity, while Steward's calculations of population density yielded a total of 2,900,000.[87] Rosenblat, whose estimate of 2,030,000 falls in between those of Kroeber and Steward, based his total on a review of the literature.[88] Denevan's first estimate, published in 1976, was 8,500,000, based on his calculations of population density, comparisons with other regions, and demographic studies of specific societies.[89] On the basis of adjusted population densities and the recent work of others, his second estimate revised this total upward to 8,620,000.[90] Following a careful review of the literature, I conclude that an estimate ranging from 7,000,000 to 8,000,000 appears reasonable.

Hemispheric Totals

Having reviewed the demographic literature on Amerindian populations in North America, Mexico, Central America, the Caribbean, the Andes, and lowland South America, we can now return to our original question, what was the size of the native population of the Americas in 1492? Estimates of the hemispheric population before contact range from 8,400,000 to 200,000,000. Because Kroeber's figures have consistently been among the lowest for all areas of the Americas, it is not surprising that his hemispheric estimate of 8,400,000 is also the smallest.[91] The highest total, 200,000,000, is also the earliest, offered by Riccioli, who in the second half of the seventeenth century published estimates of the population in various regions of the world.[92]

During the 1920s, when estimates of the native population of the Americas were in a high cycle, Rivet and Sapper both offered figures of

Date	Source	Estimate	Methodology
\multicolumn{4}{l}{Table A.7 Estimates of the Native Population of South America at Contact}
1924	Sapper	3–5,000,000	carrying capacity
1934	Kroeber	1,000,000	analogy with North America
1949	Steward	2,900,000	population density
1954	Rosenblat	2,030,000	adjusted Steward
1966	Dobyns	9–11,250,000	depopulation ratios/20:1 and 25:1
1976	Denevan	8,500,000	population density, analogy, and estimates of others
1992	Denevan	8,620,000	adjusted population densities

Table A.8 Estimates of the Native Population of the Americas at Contact			
Date	Source	Estimate	Methodology
1672	Battista Riccioli	200,000,000	guess
1924	Rivet	40–50,000,000	backward projection
1924	Sapper	40–50,000,000	carrying capacity
1928	Spinden	50–75,000,000	carrying capacity and archaeological evidence
1931	Willcox	13,111,000	based on Mooney and review of literature
1934	Kroeber	8,400,000	hemispheric—North America population ratio
1949	Steward	15,490,000	population density and adjustments to Kroeber
1954	Rosenblat	13,380,000	review of literature
1964	Borah	100,000,000	guess and carrying capacity
1966 and 1983	Dobyns	90–112,000,000	depopulation ratio/20:1 and 25:1
1967	Morner	33,300,000	reduced Borah by two-thirds
1976	Ubelaker	16,000,000	hemispheric—North America population ratio
1976	Denevan	57,300,000	based on regional totals
1987	Thornton	72,000,000	upward revision of Denevan
1992	Denevan	53,904,000	adjusted 1976 totals
1992	Whitmore	43–50,000,000	based on Denevan
1992	Stannard	75–100,000,000	review of literature

from 40,000,000 to 50,000,000, while Spinden published an estimate of from 50,000,000 to 75,000,000.[93] Then in 1931, the first of the low estimates appeared with Willcox's figure of 13,111,000, which he based on Mooney's total for North America and his own review of the literature.[94] Kroeber published his estimate of 8,400,000 three years later, followed by Steward's total of 15,490,000 in 1949. Steward based his figure on population densities and adjustments to Kroeber's work. Another low counter, Rosenblat estimated the hemispheric population at 13,380,000, based on a review of the literature.[95]

The return of the high counters began in 1964 with the publication of Woodrow Borah's estimate of 100,000,000, based both on guesswork and notions of carrying capacity.[96] Dobyns followed two years later, using depopulation ratios of 20 to 1 and 25 to 1 to arrive at a range of from 90,000,000 to 112,000,000.[97] Morner's estimate of 33,300,000 reduced Borah's figure by two-thirds but remained considerably higher than those of the low counters.[98] During the 1970s, estimates varied, ranging from Ubelaker's 16,000,000, based on adjustments to Mooney and the hemispheric–North America population ratio, to Denevan's figure of 57,300,000, based on regional totals, and Thornton's 72,000,000, an upward revision of Denevan.[99] In 1992, Denevan revised his previous estimate, adjusting it downward to 53,904,000.[100] That same year, Whitmore posited a population of from 43,000,000 to 50,000,000, based on his reading of Denevan, and Stannard based his total of 75,000,000 to 100,000,000 on a review of the literature.[101] In the popular press, estimates of from 40,000,000 to 50,000,000 have gained acceptance during the 1990s.[102] Tallying the estimates this author found most acceptable for the six regions under consideration, we arrive at a range of from 46,800,000 to 53,800,000. This falls well within the range of moderate estimates suggested originally by Rivet, Sapper, and Spinden in the 1920s and more recently by Denevan and Whitmore.

At this point, at least one thing should be clear to the reader: that historical narratives and analysis are subjective and constructed and reconstructed through argument, not, as some would believe, by the revelation of "facts." When read in isolation, both high and low counters can present their cases in ways that appear quite reasonable and convincing. In the end, it is clear that it will never be possible to know for certain how many humans lived in the Americas in 1492. And perhaps that is not what is most important anyway. According to demographic historian Robert McCaa, "What matters in history are the dynamics, not the static totals."[103] And high and low counters aside, the population dynamics of the Americas after 1492 are quite clear: native populations declined dramatically, facilitating European conquest and colonization.

· Epilogue ·

$\mathcal{A}$ small cloud of bacteria or viruses could easily and silently infect tens of thousands of people, triggering fatal outbreaks of anthrax, smallpox, pneumonic plague or any of a dozen other deadly diseases. And victims infected with contagious ailments could pass the microbes to thousands of others before doctors even figured out what was going on. Moreover, bioterrorism could foment political instability, given the panic that fast-moving plagues have historically engendered.

Rick Weiss, "Bioterrorism: An Even More Devastating Threat"

Deadly germs sprayed in shopping malls, bomblets spewing anthrax spores over battlefields, tiny vials of plague scattered in Times Square—these are the poor man's hydrogen bombs—hideous weapons of mass destruction that can be made in a simple laboratory.

Judith Miller, Steven Engleber, and William Broad, *Germs:
Biological Weapons and America's Secret War*

In order to make the ongoing story of the complex relationship between humans and disease more relevant to the reader, my original plan was to bring the story up-to-date by focusing this brief section on the outbreaks of two infectious diseases that posed serious threats to public health and claimed millions of lives during the twentieth century. These two incidents, one at the beginning of the century, the other at the end, bracketed the twentieth century and serve as grim reminders that infectious illness continues to cause enormous human suffering worldwide despite the dizzying pace of medical advances throughout this same period.

During the spring of 1918, a particularly virulent strain of influenza appeared in the United States and quickly became pandemic. While thousands died during this initial outbreak, it was subsequent waves of the disease, in the summer and fall of 1919, that proved especially lethal. And while influenza most often kills the elderly and those already weakened by other infections, in this case, more than half of the deaths were among young adults. By the time the pandemic subsided late in 1919, between 25 and 40 million people around the world had died, more than 550,000 in the United States alone. According to biological historian Alfred Crosby, "It is possible that the 1918–19 pandemic [of influenza] was, in terms of absolute numbers, the greatest single demographic shock that the human species has ever received."[1]

At the opposite end of the century, HIV-AIDS loomed as one of the greatest threats to human health. In the last two decades, this highly infectious illness has infected some 60 million people, 95 percent of whom live in the developing world. HIV-AIDS, which had claimed the lives of 2.2 million persons by 1998, is now the leading cause of death in sub-Saharan Africa and the fourth leading cause of death worldwide. Both of these pandemics, massive in both the scale and scope of their destruction, dramatically illustrate two of the central arguments of this book: that all human populations react in similar ways to the same infectious organisms and that we remain as vulnerable to the spread of infectious diseases today as our ancestors did many generations ago.

But since the destruction of the World Trade Center in New York City, the attack on the Pentagon in Washington, D.C., the hijacking and crashing of a plane in western Pennsylvania on September 11, 2001, and the now omnipresent threat of bioterrorism as evidenced most dramatically by the dissemination of anthrax, sent in letters through the U.S. postal system, this story has changed dramatically. Literally overnight, the specter of infectious disease has assumed a new relevance and urgency not previously imagined: the threat of bioterrorism and biological warfare has become terrifyingly real to people throughout the world. No longer do individuals in the United States, Western Europe, and Japan dismiss serious infectious diseases as a problem confined to the poor of the underdeveloped world; suddenly people everywhere are searching anxiously for information on anthrax, botulism, smallpox, and pneumonic plague—diseases that have been infecting human populations for centuries but that had been largely ignored, certainly in the developed world, during the last decades of the twentieth century.

By the end of World War II, the greatest fear of governments and people around the world was the proliferation of nuclear weapons and the specter of a nuclear war that would annihilate entire human populations. Since September 11, however, a new fear looms large in the minds of millions—bioterrorism. Bioterrorism is the use of, or the threatened use of, easily disseminated biological agents such as anthrax, smallpox, botulism, and pneumonic plague to intimidate or subjugate groups of people. Bioterrorism is not new: during the fourteenth and fifteenth centuries, Europeans catapulted the bodies of plague victims into the midst of their enemies in hopes of disseminating the disease. As noted above, the British attempted to spread smallpox among North American native societies by distributing blankets contaminated with scabs from victims of that dreaded disease during the eighteenth century. During World War II, the Japanese introduced plague-infected fleas into Chinese cities as part of their campaign to conquer the mainland. More recently, the government of Iraq has purportedly used biological agents against segments of its own Kurdish population.

The advantages of biological weapons are significant: First, they are inexpensive and easy to manufacture; second, their deployment does not damage valuable property as is the case in conventional or nuclear warfare; and third, because disease-causing organisms are both invisible and quiet, bioterrorism is perfectly suited to covert attacks. But biowarfare also has one major disadvantage: once released, disease agents can be unpredictable, and just as easily as they can infect the enemy, they can also reverse course and turn back on their disseminators. During World War II, the United States, Japan, Germany, and the Soviet Union all pursued covert programs in germ warfare. The government of the United States hired George Merck, the president of Merck Pharmaceuticals and a leader in the drug industry, to head the secret program, based at Camp Detrick in rural Maryland. Since that time, the governments of the United States and other nations have pursued research programs involving the use of bacterial agents such as anthrax, plague, and botulism as well as viral agents, especially smallpox. Since 1975, 143 nations have signed an international biological weapons treaty, banning the production and storage of biological weapons, but ineffectual monitoring renders the treaty virtually unenforceable.

In January 2001, the Centers for Disease Control (CDC) in Atlanta reported that the nation's public health infrastructure is not adequate to detect and respond to a bioterrorist event. Events following September 11 gave this warning new urgency, and by the end of the year, the CDC had issued information on the four infections, anthrax, botulism, pneumonic plague, and smallpox, it considered most likely to be used in acts of bioterrorism.

Anthrax is a bacterial disease that can manifest itself in three forms: cutaneous, inhalational, and gastrointestinal. Anthrax cannot be transmitted directly from person to person—rather, it occurs after individuals come into contact with the bacterial spores; symptoms usually develop within seven days following contact. While all three forms of the disease may prove fatal if left untreated, cutaneous anthrax is the least likely to result in death. Naturally occurring cutaneous anthrax occurs after contact with contaminated meat, wool, hides, or leather from infected animals, usually through a cut or abrasion on the skin. The disease often begins with a small, painless lesion on the skin, accompanied by fever, malaise, headache, and swelling of the lymph glands. This form of the disease responds well to treatment by antibiotics, but if left untreated, 20 percent mortality can be expected. Gastrointestinal anthrax is rare and usually develops following the consumption of contaminated meat.

Inhalational anthrax is the most lethal form of the disease. It occurs when an individual inhales anthrax spores directly into the lungs, producing symptoms that include sore throat, fever, muscle aches, and malaise; if not treated promptly with antibiotics, death may result from respiratory failure or meningitis.

Like anthrax, botulism cannot be transmitted directly from person to person. Rather, the disease, produced by contact with the botulinum toxin, a lethal poison produced by bacteria, can only be transmitted through contaminated food or by direct introduction into a wound. Symptoms include blurred vision, slurred speech, and difficulty with movement and breathing. Botulism quickly kills its victims by paralyzing their muscles, including those required for respiration, leading to asphyxiation.

The causes and symptoms of pneumonic plague and smallpox have both been discussed earlier in this book, but it is important to note here that both are extremely lethal infections that can be easily transmitted from person to person. It should also be noted that at the present time, there is no effective vaccine against plague. And while an effective vaccine to prevent smallpox has existed for decades, routine vaccination against the disease has been discontinued since 1972, when the World Health Organization announced that this highly contagious illness had been eradicated from human populations worldwide.

Not long after the attacks on September 11, 2001, several suspected cases of anthrax were reported to the CDC. Local and federal law enforcement agencies and public health officials quickly traced the source of infection to a series of letters that were mailed through the U.S. Postal Service. By the end of November a total of eighteen confirmed cases and five suspected cases had been documented. Of the confirmed cases, seven were diagnosed as cutaneous anthrax and eleven as inhalational. Of the eleven individuals who contracted the inhalational form of the disease, five eventually died. To date, no one has been arrested in connection with these events, but the FBI claims that a single individual, rather than an organization, is probably responsible. In addition to the suffering inflicted on the families and friends of those who contracted anthrax, the impact of this act of bioterrorism is immense. In addition to the threat of terrorist bombings and hijackings, people everywhere are now aware that they face an even more insidious threat posed by armies of invisible enemies capable of escaping the most sophisticated methods of detection.

This book, largely completed before September 11, 2001, began with the statement from medical writer Laurie Garrett that "the history of our time will be marked by recurrent eruptions of newly discovered diseases." In light of recent events, however, it appears that people in the twenty-first century remain as vulnerable to the old scourges of humankind as were their ancestors. Anthrax, botulism, plague, smallpox, and other ills have claimed the lives of many millions throughout the ages, and it appears that they are not done with us yet. In addition, we face serious threats posed by newly emerging infections such as HIV-AIDS, Ebola, and Legionnaires' disease. Thus it appears that Garrett's statement that new diseases will pose the greatest threat to human health in the twenty-first century was only partially true—present and future generations face the specter of a myriad of infections, both old and new. With respect to the ever-evolving relationship between humans and disease, the future appears uncertain at best.

• *Notes* •

Introduction

1. Stengel, "The Diffusionists Have Landed," 47.
2. Cook, *Born to Die*, 13.
3. For a more detailed discussion of The Black Legend, see ibid., 1–25.
4. Las Casas, *A Short Account*, 15.
5. Whitmore, *Disease and Death in Early Colonial Mexico*, 208.

Chapter 1

1. Cliff, *Measles: An Historical Geography*, 133–37.
2. For a discussion of the origins of a native American humoral theory see Austin Alchon, *Native Society and Disease in Colonial Ecuador*, 25–29; Foster, "On the Origin of Humoral Medicine," 355–93; and Anderson, "Why Is Humoral Medicine So Popular?" 331–37.
3. Unschuld, "History of Chinese Medicine," 24; Risse, "History of Western Medicine," 13; and Gallagher, "Islamic and Indian Medicine," 30.
4. Shigehisa, "Concepts of Disease in East Asia," 56.
5. Gottfried, *The Black Death*, 82.
6. Boccaccio, *The Decameron*, 12.
7. Austin Alchon, *Native Society and Disease in Colonial Ecuador*, 29.
8. Watts, *Epidemics in History*, 10.
9. Farris, "Diseases of the Premodern Period in Japan," 381.
10. Garcilaso de la Vega, *Royal Commentaries*, 1:413.
11. Austin Alchon, *Native Society and Disease in Colonial Ecuador*, 31.
12. Dols, *Black Death in the Middle East*, 128.
13. Ibid., 23.
14. Ibid., 62 and 157.
15. Gottfried, *The Black Death*, 84.
16. Hopkins, *Princes and Peasants*, 108.
17. McNeill, *Plagues and Peoples*, 45–46.

18. Ortner, "Diseases of the Pre-Roman World," 247–61.
19. Rhazes as cited in Hopkins, *Princes and Peasants*, 168.
20. Theal as cited in Hopkins, *Princes and Peasants*, 169.
21. Kiple, "Diseases of Sub-Saharan Africa to 1860," 293–97.
22. Chakravorty, "Diseases of Antiquity in South Asia," 408–13; and Said, "Diseases of the Premodern Period in South Asia," 413–17.
23. Wise as cited in Hopkins, *Princes and Peasants*, 16–17.
24. Ibid., 17.
25. Gwei-Djen, "Diseases of Antiquity in China," 345–54.
26. Hopkins, *Princes and Peasants*, 103–4.
27. Ibid., 109–10.
28. Farris, "Diseases of the Premodern Period in Japan," 378–81.
29. Hopkins, *Princes and Peasants*, 105–8.
30. Ortner, "Diseases of the Pre-Roman World," 258; and Stannard, "Diseases of Western Antiquity," 62–270.
31. Thucydides, *The Landmark*, 118.
32. Ibid., 120.
33. Hopkins, *Princes and Peasants*, 19–20.
34. Ibid., 22–23.
35. Ibid., 24.
36. Ibid., 26–29.
37. Carmichael and Silverstein, "Smallpox," 159.
38. Crosby, "Influenza," 808–9; and O'Neill, "Diseases of the Middle Ages," 275.
39. Moore, *The Formation of a Persecuting Society*, 48.
40. Foucault, *Madness and Civilization*, 4–5.
41. Watts, *Epidemics in History*, 44–64.
42. Ibid., 62–64; and Carmichael, "Leprosy," 839.
43. Historian David Herlihy argues against the diagnosis of bubonic plague, claiming instead that anthrax or a virulent form of tuberculosis may have been responsible for the Black Death. Herlihy, *The Black Death*, 29–30.
44. Hopkins, *Princes and Peasants*, 23.
45. Gottfried, *The Black Death*, 10–11.
46. Ibid., 11–12.
47. Benedict, *Bubonic Plague in Nineteenth-Century China*, 9–10.
48. Said, "Diseases of the Premodern Period in South Asia," 415–16.
49. See Benedict, *Bubonic Plague in Nineteenth-Century China*, 10.
50. Park, "Black Death," 612–13.
51. Herlihy, *The Black Death*, 17.
52. Watts, *Epidemics in History*, 25–26.
53. Carmichael, *Plague and the Poor*, 108–26; and Watts, *Epidemics in History*, 15–25.
54. Watts, *Epidemics in History*, 25–39.
55. Herlihy, "The Bright Side of the Plague," 26.
56. Duncan-Jones, "The Impact of the Antonine Plague," 111.
57. Farris, "Diseases of the Premodern Period in Japan," 378–81.
58. Gottfried, *Epidemic Disease in Fifteenth Century England*, 47–50.
59. McNeill, *Plagues and Peoples*, 116–25 and 260–69.

Chapter 2

1. Begley and Murr, "The First Americans," 50–57.
2. Stengel, "The Diffusionists Have Landed," 35–48.
3. Guaman Poma de Ayala, *La nueva corónica y buen gobierno*, 1:89.
4. Roys, *The Book of Chilam Balam of Chumayel*, 83.
5. Nabokov, *Native American Testimony*, 25.
6. According to Kirkpatrick Sale, "One reason that the Indian populations, in the Caribbean as elsewhere, were so vulnerable to diseases of any kind [after 1492] is that, to an extraordinary extent, the Americas were free of any serious pathogens. The presumed passage of the original Indian populations across the Bering Strait tens of thousands of years before served to freeze to death most human disease carriers except a few intestinal ones, it is thought, and there were apparently none established on the continents previously, so in general the Indians enjoyed remarkably good health, free of both endemic and epidemic scourges." Sale, *The Conquest of Paradise*, 160. See also Ortiz de Montellano, *Aztec Medicine, Health, and Nutrition*, 120; Dobyns, *Their Number Become Thinned*, 34; Thornton, *American Indian Holocaust and Survival*, 39; Austin Alchon, *Native Society and Disease in Colonial Ecuador*, 19–31; and Newson, *Life and Death in Early Colonial Ecuador*, 144.
7. Guaman Poma de Ayala, *Letter to a King*, 26, 40, 42.
8. Sahagún, *Florentine Codex*, 9:2.
9. Larsen, "In the Wake of Columbus," 115 and 125.
10. Storey, *Life and Death in the Ancient City of Teotihuacan*, 238–66.
11. Ortner, "Skeletal Paleopathology," 7.
12. Kiple, "Skeletal Biology and the History of Native Americans and African Americans," 3–10; and Larsen, "In the Wake of Columbus," 116.
13. Jaffee, *The First Immigrants from Asia*, 58; and Cassidy, "Skeletal Evidence for Prehistoric Subsistence Adaptation," 320.
14. Dunn, "Epidemiological Factors: Health and Disease in Hunter-Gatherers," 223–24; Buikstra, "Diseases of the Pre-Columbian Americas," 305; and Jaffee, *The First Immigrants from Asia*, 58–60.
15. Jaffee, *The First Immigrants from Asia*, 60.
16. Larsen, "In the Wake of Columbus," 118–19.
17. Ibid.
18. Dunn, "Epidemiological Factors: Health and Disease in Hunter-Gatherers," 224–25.
19. Austin Alchon, *Native Society and Disease in Colonial Ecuador*, 23.
20. Merbs, "A New World of Infectious Disease," 15.
21. Allison, "Paleopathology in Peruvian and Chilean Populations," 520–21.
22. Buikstra, "Diseases of the Pre-Columbian Americas," 310.
23. Allison, "Paleopathology in Peruvian and Chilean Populations," 520–21.
24. Buikstra, "Diseases of the Pre-Columbian Americas," 311.
25. McGrath, "A Computer Simulation of the Spread of Tuberculosis in Prehistoric Populations of the Lower Illinois River Valley."
26. Armelagos, "Health and Disease in Prehistoric Populations in Transition," 130.
27. Milner, "Disease and Sociopolitical Systems in Late Prehistoric Illinois," 105.

28. Stodder and Martin, "Health and Disease in the Southwest Before and After Spanish Contact," 61.
29. Larsen, "In the Wake of Columbus," 117.
30. Storey, *Life and Death in the Ancient City of Teotihuacan,* 230–31; and McCaa, "Paradise, Hells, and Purgatories," 6–7.
31. Larsen, "Health and Disease in Prehistoric Georgia," 374–79.
32. Kiple, "Skeletal Biology and the History of Native Americans and African Americans," 6; Armelagos, "Health and Disease in Prehistoric Populations," 137–40; and Goodman, et al., "Health Changes at Dickson Mounds, Illinois," 297.
33. Armelagos, "Paleopathology in Peruvian and Chilean Populations," 138–39.
34. Bollet and Brown, "Anemia," 572–73.
35. McCaa, "Paradise, Hells, and Purgatories," 8.
36. Jaffee, *The First Immigrants from Asia,* 58; Cook, "Subsistence and Health in the Lower Illinois Valley," 261; and Cohen, "Paleopathology at the Origins of Agriculture: Editors' Summation," 592.
37. Allison, "Paleopathology in Peruvian and Chilean Populations," 525–26; and Verano, "Prehistoric Disease and Demography in the Andes," 21.
38. Storey, *Life and Death in the Ancient City of Teotihuacan,* 184–85. In sharp contrast to the short life expectancies of native Americans posited by these studies, two paleopathologists claim, "In many of the 23 pre-Columbian cultures we have studied, at least 40% of the population lived past the age of 40 years, including them in a geriatric population. Many of these cultures had a geriatric survival rate of greater than 25%." Unfortunately, the authors do not give citations for their findings, nor do they offer further explanations. See Gerszten and Allison, "Human Soft Tissue Tumors in Paleopathology," 259.
39. Russell, *Late Ancient and Medieval Population,* 75 and 175; and Duncan-Jones, "The Impact of the Antonine Plague," 116.
40. Buikstra, "Tuberculosis in the Americas," 165.
41. Allison, "Paleopathology in Peruvian and Chilean Populations," 521.
42. Zinsser, *Rats, Lice and History,* 236.
43. Guaman Poma de Ayala, *Letter to a King,* 42.
44. Ibid., 77.
45. Cook, "The Incidence and Significance of Disease Among the Aztecs and Related Tribes," 320–35; and Roys, *The Book of Chilam Balam of Chumayel,* 133 and 142.
46. Merbs, "A New World of Infectious Disease," 27; Ortiz de Montellano, *Aztec Medicine, Health, and Nutrition,* 121; Cook, "The Incidence and Significance of Disease Among the Aztecs and Related Tribes," 321–22. All of the aforementioned claim that typhus was not present in the Americas before 1492. Zinsser, *Rats, Lice and History,* 253–64; Hernández, "Epidemias y calamides en el Mexico prehispanico," 215–31; Fernandez, "El tifus en Mexico antes de Zinsser," 127; and León, "Que era el Matlazahuatl y que el cocoliztli en los tiempos precolumbinos y en la epoca hispana?" 385. These four authors argue that typhus was present in the New World before the arrival of Europeans.

47. MacLeod, *Spanish Central America*, 19; Cook, "The Incidence and Significance of Disease Among the Aztecs and Related Tribes," 321; Veblen, "Native Population Decline in Totonicapan, Guatemala," 484–99; and Gerhard, *A Guide to the Historical Geography of New Spain*, 23.
48. Flores as cited in Cook, "The Incidence and Significance of Disease Among the Aztecs and Related Tribes," 321.
49. Ibid., 330.
50. Ibid., 333–35; and Hernández, "Epidemias y calamides en el Mexico pre-hispano," 129.
51. Saunders, Ramsden, and Herring, "Transformation and Disease: Precontact Ontario Iroquoians," 121.
52. Smith, "Virus Spreading by Ducks Spurs Immunologists," 1–2.
53. Crosby, "Influenza," 808.
54. Merbs, "A New World of Infectious Disease," 35; and Newman, "Aboriginal New World Epidemiology," 669.
55. Patterson, *Pandemic Influenza*, 5–6.
56. Roys, *The Book of Chilam Balam of Chumayel*, 103, 115, and 133–34.
57. Ibid., 133.
58. Ibid.
59. Salomon, *The Huarochiri Manuscript*, 5, 361, 377, and 468.
60. Duran, *The History of the Indies of New Spain*, 238–41; Sahagún, *Florentine Codex*, 9:2; and Cook, "The Incidence and Significance of Disease Among the Aztecs and Related Tribes," 330–35.
61. Cook, "The Incidence and Significance of Disease Among the Aztecs and Related Tribes," 331.
62. Duran, *The History of the Indies of New Spain*, 240.
63. Larsen, "In the Wake of Columbus," 117–19.
64. Cieza de León, *Obras completas*, 1:53.
65. Ibid., 1:224.
66. Jimenez de la Espada, *Relaciones geográficas*, 2:267.
67. Larsen, "In the Wake of Columbus," 117–19.

Chapter 3

1. Cook, "Disease and Depopulation of Hispaniola, 1492–1518," 220–28.
2. Guerra, "La epidemia americana de influenza en 1493," 325–47; and Cook, "Disease and Depopulation of Hispaniola, 1492–1518," 227.
3. Las Casas, *Historia de las Indias*, 1:419–20.
4. Cook, "Disease and Depopulation of Hispaniola, 1492–1518," 228–31.
5. Ibid., 232–33.
6. Ibid., 233–35.
7. Ibid., 232–36.
8. Las Casas, *Historia de las Indias*, 3:270.
9. Fernandez de Oviedo, *Historia general*, 1:105.
10. *Colección de documentos inéditos*, 1:367–68 and 369–70.
11. Ibid., 1:397–98.
12. Las Casas, *Historia de las Indias*, 2:257; and Fernandez de Oviedo, *Historia general*, 1:105.
13. Landa, *Landa's relación de las cosas de Yucatán*, 41; and Roys, *The Book of Chilam Balam of Chumayel*, 138 and 205.

14. Vázquez de Ayllón, as cited in McCaa, "Spanish and Nahuatl Views," 402–4.
15. Sahagún, *Florentine Codex*, 13:81.
16. Cortés, *Letters from Mexico*, 164.
17. While most scholars agree that introduction of smallpox to Mexico in 1520 produced devastating demographic consequences, historian Francis J. Brooks disagrees, claiming that the epidemic was "a mild attack of smallpox, such as occurred in contemporary Europe with some suffering, some deaths, and little further effect." He added that no demographic catastrophe occurred. Brooks, "Revising the Conquest of Mexico," 1–29.
18. McCaa, "Spanish and Nahuatl Views," 400–401.
19. Motolinia o Benavente, *Memoriales*, 294; and Vázquez, *Relación*, 148.
20. McBryde, "Influenza in America," 296–302; Feldman, "Active Measures in the War Against Epidemics," 1–11; and Lovell, *Conquest and Survival*, 70.
21. Recinos and Goetz, eds., *Annals of the Cakchiquels*, 115–16.
22. "Instrucciones a los procuradores . . . ," as cited in Newson, *The Cost of Conquest*, 128, n. 50.
23. Reff, *Disease, Depopulation, and Culture Change*, 99–103.
24. Crosby, "Conquistador y pestilencia," 321–37; Dobyns, *Their Number Become Thinned*, 12; McNeill, *Plagues and Peoples*, 207.
25. Garcilaso de la Vega, *Royal Commentaries*, 572–78.
26. Cabello de Balboa, *Miscelanea Antartica*, 393; and Sarmiento de Gamboa, *Historia de los Incas*, 148.
27. Cieza de León, *Obras completas*, 1:219.
28. Cobo, *History of the Inca Empire*, 160–61.
29. Santa Cruz Pachacuti, *Relación*, 36; and Guaman Poma de Ayala, *La nueva corónica*, 1:85 and 207.
30. Measles is characterized by a rash that appears first on the face. In smallpox, the rash that appears initially evolves into pustules, eventually forming scabs.
31. Motolinia o Benavente, *Memoriales*, 22. While Motolinia labeled the disease as *sarampion*, or measles, historian Hanns Prem argues that a description of high child mortality militates against this diagnosis. If the illness had been measles, all segments of the population, not just children, would be expected to succumb. For similar reasons, Prem also discounts smallpox, chicken pox, and scarlet fever as possible causes. He concludes that it is impossible to offer a reliable diagnosis of the disease responsible for the epidemic of 1531. Prem, "Disease Outbreaks in Central Mexico," 27–30.
32. Borah as cited in Cook, "Impact of Disease in the Sixteenth-Century Andean World," 208.
33. Cieza de León, *Obras completas*, 1:219.
34. See note 31.
35. Prem, "Disease Outbreaks in Central Mexico," 30–31.
36. Motolinia o Benavente, *Memoriales*, 413.
37. Prem, "Disease Outbreaks in Central Mexico," 31–34.
38. Ibid., 34–35.
39. Ibid., 35–38.
40. Paso y Troncoso, *Epistolario*, 12:86.

41. Gerhard, *A Guide to the Historical Geography of New Spain,* 23.

42. Prem, "Disease Outbreaks in Central Mexico," 38–42.

43. Gerhard, *A Guide to the Historical Geography of New Spain,* 23; and Malvido, "Cronología de epidemias," 1:172–74.

44. McCaa, "Spanish and Nahuatl Views," 429–31.

45. Lovell, "Disease in Early Colonial Guatemala," 49–83.

46. Archivo General de Indias (AGI), Guatemala 9A, as cited in Lovell, "Disease in Early Colonial Guatemala," 70.

47. Lovell, "Disease in Early Colonial Guatemala," 71–72.

48. AGI, Justicia 299, as cited in Lovell, "Disease in Early Colonial Guatemala," 71.

49. Fuentes y Guzman, *Recordación Florida,* 3:426; MacLeod, *Spanish Central America,* 98; and Orellana, *Indian Medicine,* 143, 146.

50. Recinos and Goetz, eds., *Annals of the Cakchiquels,* 143–44.

51. Martinez Duran, *Las ciencias médicas,* 79–80; Figueroa Marroquin, *Enfermedades de los conquistadores,* 57.

52. McBryde, "Influenza in America," 296–302.

53. Lovell, "Disease in Early Colonial Guatemala," 75–77.

54. Newson, "The Depopulation of Nicaragua," 278.

55. Ibid., 279; Newson, *The Cost of Conquest,* 128; and MacLeod, *Spanish Central America,* 98.

56. Porras Barrenecha, *Cartas del Peru,* 22.

57. Herrera y Tordesillas, *Historia general,* 10:72.

58. Newson, "The Depopulation of Nicaragua," 280; and Newson, *The Cost of Conquest,* 129.

59. Newson, "The Depopulation of Nicaragua," 280.

60. Newson, *The Cost of Conquest,* 129.

61. Lovell and Lutz, *Demography and Empire,* 6; and Newson, *Indian Survival in Colonial Nicaragua,* 339.

62. Newson, *The Cost of Conquest,* 331.

63. Cieza de León, *Obras completas,* 1:36.

64. Zinsser, *Rats, Lice and History,* 256; McNeill, *Plagues and Peoples,* 209; and Dobyns, "An Outline of Andean Epidemic History," 499–500. Subsequently Dobyns has written that the epidemic of 1546 may have been bubonic plague. Dobyns, *Their Number Become Thinned,* 264–65.

65. Newson and MacLeod both believe that the 1545–1546 epidemics in Mexico and Peru were attributable to pneumonic plague. Newson, "Old World Epidemics," 95–96; and MacLeod, *Spanish Central America,* 119; Cook cites plague as well as typhus. Cook, *Demographic Collapse,* 68 and 71.

66. "La ciudad de Quito," in Jimenez de la Espada, *Relaciones geográficas,* 3:205.

67. Dobyns, *Their Number Become Thinned,* 269–70.

68. Kilbourne, *Influenza,* 157–228.

69. Cook, *Demographic Collapse,* 70.

70. Toribio Polo, "Apuntes sobre las epidemias," 58.

71. Dobyns, "An Outline of Andean Epidemic History," 501.

72. It is also possible that the disease was introduced by slaves coming from the Cape Verde Islands. Dobyns, "An Outline of Andean Epidemic History," 503–4.

73. Ibid., 504.
74. Ibid., 503–5.
75. Levillier, *Gobernantes del Peru*, 11:207–8.
76. Ibid., 11:221–22.
77. Ibid., 11:284–85.
78. Paredes Borja, *Historia de la medicina*, 1:254.
79. AGI, Quito 23, as cited in Austin Alchon, *Native Society and Disease in Colonial Ecuador*, 42, n. 41.
80. Austin Alchon, *Native Society and Disease in Colonial Ecuador*, 130; Newson, *Life and Death in Early Colonial Ecuador*, 340; and Cook, *Demographic Collapse*, 94.
81. Newson, *Life and Death in Early Colonial Ecuador*, 256 and 346.
82. Ibid., 277–78, 287, 294.
83. Ibid., 311 and 323.
84. Cieza de León, *Obras completas*, 2:127; Friede, "Demographic Changes in the Mining Community of Muzo," 339; and Villamarin, "Epidemic Disease," 114.
85. Cieza de León, *Obras completas*, 1:48.
86. Villamarin, *Indian Labor*, 80–92.
87. Dixon, *Smallpox*, 325; and Fenner, *Smallpox and Its Eradication*, 175.
88. López de Gómara, *Cortés*, 204–5.
89. Sahagún, *Historia general*, 791.
90. Motolinia o Benavente, *Memoriales*, 294.

Chapter 4

1. Dean, "Indigenous Populations of the São Paulo–Rio de Janeiro Coast," 10.
2. Ibid., 11.
3. Ibid.
4. Staden, *Hans Staden: The True Story of His Captivity*, 85–89.
5. Hemming, *Red Gold*, 140.
6. Ibid., 141; and Dean, "Indigenous Populations of the São Paulo–Rio de Janeiro Coast," 21.
7. Hemming, *Red Gold*, 140.
8. Ibid., 142.
9. Ibid.
10. Ibid., 143–44.
11. Ibid., 144.
12. Ibid., 144–45.
13. Ibid., 175.
14. Ibid., 169.
15. Alden and Miller, "Out of Africa," 195–224.
16. Hemming, *Red Gold*, 338–39.
17. Alden and Miller, "Out of Africa," 203.
18. Hemming, *Red Gold*, 467–68.
19. Dean, "Indigenous Populations of the São Paulo–Rio de Janeiro Coast," 23
20. Seaver, *The Frozen Echo*, 59–60.
21. Hariot, *A Briefe and True Report*, 1:378.
22. Milanich, *Florida Indians and the Invasion from Europe*, 111.
23. Dobyns, *Their Number Become Thinned*, 270 and 275–90.

24. Larsen, et al., "Population Decline and Extinction in La Florida," 27.
25. Milanich, *Florida Indians and the Invasion from Europe*, 214–18.
26. Hann, *Apalachee*, 175.
27. Ibid., 23 and 176–77.
28. Ibid., 163.
29. Dobyns, *Their Number Become Thinned*, 288.
30. Milanich, *Florida Indians and the Invasion from Europe*, 221–31.
31. Ramenofsky, *Vectors of Death*, 71; and Milner, "Epidemic Disease in the Postcontact Southeast," 39–56.
32. Bourne, *Narratives of the Career of Hernando de Soto*, 1:66.
33. Garcilaso de la Vega, *The Florida of the Inca*, 325.
34. St Cosme, "Letter to the Bishop of Quebec," 72.
35. Du Pratz, *The History of Louisiana*, 292
36. Milner, "Epidemic Disease in Postcontact Southeast," 46; Duffy, *Epidemics in Colonial America*, 71–72.
37. Wood, "The Changing Population of the Colonial South," 89–90.
38. Reff, *Disease, Depopulation, and Culture Change*, 99–114.
39. Tello as cited in Reff, *Disease, Depopulation, and Culture Change*, 250–51.
40. Ibid., 114–17.
41. Ibid., 119–32.
42. Ibid., 135.
43. Ibid., 132–79.
44. Stodder and Martin, "Health and Disease in the Southwest Before and After Spanish Contact," 66.
45. Ibid., 66–67.
46. Ibid.
47. Snow and Lamphear, "European Contact and Indian Depopulation," 18.
48. Carlson, "Impact of Disease on Populations of New England," 147.
49. Biard as cited in Thwaites, *Jesuit Relations*, 3:105.
50. Ibid., 1:177.
51. Adams, *Three Episodes in Massachusetts History*, 1:11.
52. Ibid., 1:10–11.
53. Bratton, "The Identity of the New England Indian Epidemic of 1616–19," 351–83.
54. Adams, *Three Episodes in Massachusetts History*, 1:9.
55. Ibid., 1:12.
56. Bradford, *History of Plymouth Plantation*, 2:193–94.
57. Cook, "The Significance of Disease in the Extinction of the New England Indian," 493.
58. Ibid., 493–95.
59. Ibid., 493; and Duffy, *Epidemics in Colonial America*, 43–69.
60. Cook, "The Significance of Disease in the Extinction of the New England Indian," 501; and Snow and Lamphear, "European Contact and Indian Depopulation," 28.
61. Hudson as cited in Walker, et al., "The Effects of European Contact on the Health of Alta California Indians," 419.
62. Walker and Johnson, "Effects of Contact on the Chumash Indians," 129.

63. Ibid., 133–35; and Walker and Johnson, "The Decline of the Chumash Indian Population," 110–14.
64. Cook, "The Conflict between the California Indian and White Civilization," 5.
65. Walker and Johnson, "Effects of Contact on the Chumash Indians," 136.
66. Maud as cited in Harris, "Voices of Disaster," 596.
67. T. Manby Journal, December 1790–June 1793, William Robertson Coe Collection, Yale University, 43.
68. Harris, "Voices of Disaster," 600.
69. Ibid., 601.
70. Ibid., 604–5.
71. Boyd, "Commentary of Early Contact-Era Smallpox," 308–9.
72. Ibid., 309.
73. Boyd, "Population Decline from Two Epidemics on the Northwest Coast," 250.
74. Campbell, *Post-Columbian Culture History in the Northern Columbia Plateau*, 186.
75. Vibert, "The Natives Were Strong to Live," 207–10.
76. Harris, "Voices of Disaster," 618; and Cybulski, "Culture Change, Demographic History, and Health and Disease on the Northwest Coast," 80.
77. Sundstrom, "Smallpox Used Them Up," 305–43.
78. Ramenofsky, *Vectors of Death*, 123–24; Owsley, "Demography of Prehistoric and Early Historic Northern Plains Populations," 83; and Jantz and Owsley, "White Traders in the Upper Missouri," 189–99.
79. Nasatir, *Before Lewis and Clark*, 1:299.
80. Reinhard, "Trade, Contact, and Female Health in Northeast Nebraska," 65.
81. Chardon, *Chardon's Journal at Fort Clark*, 138–39.
82. Ibid., 124–25 and 129.
83. Trimble, "The 1837–38 Smallpox Epidemic on the Upper Missouri," 82–84.
84. Reff, *Disease, Depopulation, and Culture Change*, 207–9.

Chapter 5

1. Bastien, *Healers of the Andes*, 46.
2. Garcilaso de la Vega, *Royal Commentaries*, 1:122.
3. Lopez Austin, *The Human Body*, 1:274.
4. Ibid., 1:259, 272, 274.
5. Pires as cited in Hemming, *Red Gold*, 140.
6. Hariot, *A Briefe and True Report*, 378–79.
7. Fenn, "Biological Warfare Circa 1750," 25.
8. Spalding, *Huarochirí*, 247.
9. Blasques as cited in Hemming, *Red Gold*, 141.
10. Frontenac as cited in Bailey, *The Conflict of European and Eastern Algonkian Cultures*, 78.
11. Munoz Camargo as cited in McCaa, "Spanish and Nahuatl Views," 421.
12. Stocklein as cited in Stearn and Stearn, *The Effect of Smallpox on the Destiny of the American Indian*, 17.

13. Hemming, *Red Gold,* 338.
14. Chardon, *Chardon's Journal at Fort Clark,* 132.
15. Las Casas, *A Short Account,* 29–30.
16. Cook, *Born to Die,* 128.
17. Du Pratz, *The History of Louisiana,* 305–6.
18. Chardon, *Chardon's Journal at Fort Clark,* 129, 131, 133.
19. Dobyns, *Their Number Become Thinned,* 256.
20. Hemming, *Red Gold,* 156–57.
21. Stern, *Peru's Indian Peoples,* 51.
22. Ibid., 188.
23. Vibert, "The Natives Were Strong to Live," 221.
24. Thornton, *We Shall Live Again,* 46.
25. Ibid., 47.
26. Las Casas, *Historia de las Indias,* 3:270.
27. Motolinia o Benavente, *Memoriales,* 22.
28. Boyd, "Population Decline from Two Epidemics on the Northwest Coast," 50–51.
29. Anchieta as cited in Hemming, *Red Gold,* 142.
30. Cook, *Born to Die,* 119.
31. Garcilaso de la Vega, *Royal Commentaries,* 1:120–2.
32. Chardon, *Chardon's Journal at Fort Clark,* 130–31.
33. Ibid., 127.
34. Lery, *History of a Voyage,* 172.
35. Chardon, *Chardon's Journal at Fort Clark,* 132.
36. Hernández, *Obras completas,* 5:425.
37. Arriaga, *Extirpation,* 71.
38. Cook, *Born to Die,* 188.
39. Austin Alchon, *Native Society and Disease in Colonial Ecuador,* 72.
40. "Virrey Conde del Villar a los medicos y oficiales del Virreinato del Peru" (1589).
41. Estrada Ycaza, *El hospital,* 6.
42. Ibid.
43. Astudillo Espinosa, *Páginas históricas,* 57.
44. Chardon, *Chardon's Journal at Fort Clark,* 133.
45. Bradford, *History of Plymouth Plantation,* 2:194.
46. Frost, "The Pueblo Indian Smallpox Epidemic in New Mexico, 1898–1899," 437–40.
47. Bradford, *History of Plymouth Plantation,* 2:194.
48. Frost, "The Pueblo Indian Smallpox Epidemic in New Mexico, 1898–1899," 437.
49. Watts, *Epidemics in History,* 2–3.
50. Newson, *The Cost of Conquest,* 127–28.
51. Cieza de León, *The Discovery and Conquest of Peru,* 213.
52. Lovell, *Conquest and Survival,* 58–69.
53. Reff, *Disease, Depopulation, and Culture Change,* 114.
54. Cortés, *Cartas,* 109.
55. Ibid., 116.
56. Díaz del Castillo, *The Conquest of Mexico,* 405–6.
57. Austin Alchon, *Native Society and Disease in Colonial Ecuador,* 34.

58. Austin Alchon, "Indians, Conquistadors, and Land," 5.
59. Burkholder and Johnson, *Colonial Latin America*, 114.
60. Hemming, *Red Gold*, 147.
61. Ibid., 148.
62. Ibid., 175.
63. Ibid., 171–72.
64. Ibid., 174–75.
65. Fieldhouse, *Colonial Empires*, 35–37.
66. Nester, *The Great Frontier War*, 15 and 60.
67. Seed, *Ceremonies of Possession*, 65.
68. Nester, *The Great Frontier War*, 2.
69. Ibid., 18.
70. Sleeper-Smith, "Women, Kin and Catholicism," 436.
71. Nester, *The Great Frontier War*, 14.
72. Ibid., 16.
73. Seed, *Ceremonies of Possession*, 19.
74. Ibid., 39.
75. Pagden, *Lords of All the World*, 37.
76. Nester, *The Great Frontier War*, 7.
77. Ibid., 11.
78. Ibid., 13.
79. Oberg, *Dominion and Civility*, 239.
80. Nester, *The Great Frontier War*, 13.
81. Ibid., 2.
82. Newson, *The Cost of Conquest*, 107–11.
83. Newson, *Indian Survival in Colonial Nicaragua*, 118.
84. Hemming, *Red Gold*, 149.
85. Ibid., 147.
86. Ibid., 151.
87. Ibid., 143 and 152.
88. Ibid., 150 and 156.
89. Miller, *Skyscrapers Hide the Heavens*, 54.
90. Duncan, "Indian Slavery," 86–91.
91. Ibid., 92.
92. Ibid., 98–99.
93. Newson, *The Cost of Conquest*, 203.
94. Powers, *Andean Journeys*, 45.
95. Ibid., 13–43.
96. Johnson, "Portuguese Settlement," 24.
97. Watts, *Epidemics in History*, 2 and 26.
98. Stengel, "The Diffusionists Have Landed," 46.

Appendix
1. Osborne, "The Numbers Game," 53.
2. Henige, "Native American Population at Contact," 2–23.
3. Rivet and Loukotka, "Langues americaines," 597–712; Sapper, "Die Zahl und die Volksdichte der indianischen Bevolkerung in America," 1:95–104; and Spinden, "The Population of Ancient America," 641–60.

4. Kroeber, "Native American Population," 1–25; and Rosenblat, "El desarrollo de la población indígena de América," 1(1):115–33, 1(2):117–48, and 1(3):109–41.
5. Cook and Borah, *The Aboriginal Population of Central Mexico in the Sixteenth Century.*
6. Morner, *Race Mixture in the History of Latin America,* 12; and Dobyns, "Reassessing New World Populations at the Time of Contact."
7. Cook and Borah, "Materials for the Demographic History of Mexico, 1500–1960," 1:13.
8. Cook and Borah, *The Aboriginal Population of Central Mexico in the Sixteenth Century.*
9. Cook and Borah, "The Aboriginal Population of Hispaniola," 1:376–410.
10. Cook, *Demographic Collapse,* 59–74.
11. Henige, *Numbers from Nowhere,* 88–112.
12. Cortés's comments regarding the size of native populations and other matters are contained in a series of letters he wrote to the king of Spain. See Cortés, *Cartas.*
13. Phelan, *The Kingdom of Quito,* 44; Tyrer, "The Demographic and Economic History of the Audiencia of Quito," 3–4; Austin Alchon, *Native Society and Disease in Colonial Ecuador,* 12–18; Newson, *Life and Death in Early Colonial Ecuador,* 58–60.
14. Henige, *Numbers from Nowhere,* 304.
15. Riccioli, *Geographiae Hydrographiae Reformatae,* 679–80.
16. Rosenblat, *La población indígena,* 1:102; and Steward, "The Native Population of South America," 5:655–68.
17. Kroeber, "Native American Population," 25.
18. Dobyns, *Their Number Become Thinned,* 37–42.
19. Cook, *Demographic Collapse,* 59–74.
20. Zambardino, "Review of Noble David Cook, *Demographic Collapse,*" 719–22.
21. Dobyns, "Estimating Aboriginal American Population," 415.
22. Cook, *Demographic Collapse,* 14–29.
23. Crosby, "Summary on Population Size before and after Contact," 277–78.
24. Ramenofsky, *Vectors of Death,* 42–71.
25. Zambardino, "Critique of David Henige's 'On the Contact Population of Hispaniola': History as Higher Mathematics," 700–712; and Whitmore, *Disease and Death in Early Colonial Mexico,* 3.
26. Stannard, *American Indian Holocaust,* 263–28.
27. Stiffarm and Lane, "The Demography of Native North America: A Question of American Indian Survival," 28–31.
28. Dobyns, *Their Number Become Thinned,* 37–42.
29. Ibid., 42.
30. Kroeber, "Native American Population," 1–25; and Mooney, *The Aboriginal Population of America North of Mexico.*
31. Ubelaker, "The Sources and Methodology for Mooney's Estimates of North American Indian Populations," 243–88.
32. Ubelaker, "Prehistoric New World Population Size," 661.
33. Sapper, "Die Zahl und die Volksdichte der indianischen Bevölkerung in America," 1:95–104; and MacLeod, *The American Indian Frontier,* 15–16.

34. Dobyns, "Estimating Aboriginal American Population," 395–416.
35. Driver, *Indians of North America*, 63–65.
36. Ubelaker, "Prehistoric New World Population Size," 661–65.
37. Denevan, *The Native Population of the Americas in 1492* (1976): 291.
38. Hughes, *American Indian Ecology*, 95–104.
39. Thornton, *American Indian Holocaust*, 32.
40. Ramenofsky, *Vectors of Death*, 160–62.
41. Ubelaker, "North American Indian Population Size," 289–94.
42. Denevan, *The Native Population of the Americas in 1492* (1992): xxviii.
43. Díaz del Castillo, *The Conquest of Mexico*, 216.
44. Cortés, *Letters from Mexico*, 102–3.
45. Kroeber, "Native American Population," 21.
46. Sapper, "Die Zahl und die Volksdichte der indianischen Bevolkerung in America," 1:12–16.
47. Steward, "The Native Population of South America," 5:655–68; and Rosenblat, *La población indígena*, 1:102.
48. Cook and Borah, *The Aboriginal Population of Central Mexico on the Eve of the Spanish Conquest*.
49. Dobyns, "Estimating Aboriginal American Population," 395–416.
50. Ibid., 395–416; and "Reassessing New World Populations," 8–9.
51. Responding to Dobyns's figure of 30,000,000 to 37,500,000, Driver argued that this was too high and that 20,000,000, the size of Mexico's population in 1940, might better represent the pre-Columbian demographic situation. Driver, *Indians of North America*, 63–64; Denevan's total of 21,400,000 was based on the average of Cook and Borah's 25,200,000 and Sander's 11,400,000 for central Mexico with additions for regions outside the central area. Denevan, "Epilogue" (1976): 289–92; Slicher von Bath adjusted the conversion factor of tributaries to total population, thus reducing Cook and Borah's total by 15 percent to 21,420,000. Slicher von Bath, "The Calculation of the Population of New Spain, Especially for the Period before 1570," 67–95.
52. Sanders, *The Teotihuacan Valley Project, Final Report*, 1:385–457.
53. Denevan, *The Native Population of the Americas in 1492* (1976):81.
54. Zambardino, "Errors in Historical Demography," 240.
55. Whitmore, "A Simulation of the Sixteenth-Century Population Collapse in the Basin of Mexico," 477.
56. Denevan, *The Native Population of the Americas in 1492* (1992): xxviii.
57. Kroeber, "Native American Population," 21–23; and Rosenblat, *La población indígena*, 1:102.
58. Dobyns, "Estimating Aboriginal American Population," 414–15.
59. Sapper, "Die Zahl und die Volksdichte der indianischen Bevolkerung in America," 1:95–104.
60. Steward, "The Native Population of South America," 5:655–68.
61. Driver, *Indians of North America*, 64.
62. Denevan, "Epilogue" (1976): 291.
63. Sherman, *Forced Native Labor in Sixteenth-Century Central America*, 5 and 347–55.
64. Denevan, *The Native Population of the Americas in 1492* (1992): xxviii.
65. Lovell, *Demography and Empire*, 4–5.

66. Verlinden, "La population de L'Amerique précolumbienne," 453–62.
67. Cook, "The Aboriginal Population of Hispaniola," 1:376–410.
68. Henige, "On the Contact Population of Hispaniola," 232.
69. Las Casas, *Historia de las Indias*, 2:51–2 and 217.
70. Las Casas, "Memorial to Cardinal Ximenz de Cisneros," 1:255.
71. Zuazo in *Colección de documentos inéditos*, 1:310; Santo Domingo as reported by Las Casas, *Historia de las Indias*, 2:397; and Anghiera, *Décadas del Nuevo Mundo*, 273.
72. Federman as cited in Rodríguez Demorizi, *Los domínicos y las encomiendas de indios*, 19.
73. Rosenblat, "The Population of Hispaniola," 43–66.
74. Moya Pons, *La Española en el siglo XVI*, 67; and Moya Pons, *Después de Colón*, 181–89.
75. Zambardino, "Critique of David Henige's 'On the Contact Population of Hispaniola': History as Higher Mathematics," 700–708.
76. Denevan, *The Native Population of the Americas in 1492* (1992): xxviii and 291.
77. Cook, "Disease and the Depopulation of Hispaniola," 213–45.
78. Kroeber, "Native American Population," 24; and Denevan, "Epilogue" (1976): 291.
79. Steward, "The Native Population of South America," 5:655–68; and Rosenblat, *La población indígena*, 1:102.
80. Dobyns, "Estimating Aboriginal American Population," 415.
81. Sapper, "Die Zahl und die Volksdichte der indianischen Bevolkerung in America," 1:95–104.
82. Denevan, *The Native Population of the Americas in 1492* (1992): xxviii.
83. Kroeber, "Native American Population," 24; Rowe, "Inca Culture at the Time of the Spanish Conquest," 2:185; Steward, "The Native Population of South America," 5:656; Rosenblat, *La población indígena*, 1:102; Shea, "A Defense of Small Population Estimates for the Central Andes in 1520," 157–80; Zambardino, "Review of Noble David Cook, *Demographic Collapse*," 719–22.
84. Sapper, "Die Zahl und die Volksdichte der indianischen Bevolkerung in America," 1:95–104; Dobyns, "Estimating Aboriginal American Population," 45; Denevan, *The Native Population of the Americas in 1492* (1976): xxviii and 291; Smith, "Depopulation of the Central Andes," 453–64; Wachtel, *Vision of the Vanquished*, 90; and Cook, *Demographic Collapse*, 23–24.
85. Verano, "Prehistoric Disease and Demography in the Andes," 16.
86. Kroeber, "Native American Population," 24; and Dobyns, "Estimating Aboriginal American Population," 414–15.
87. Sapper, "Die Zahl und die Volksdichte der indianischen Bevolkerung in America," 1:95–104; and Steward, "The Native Population of South America," 5:656.
88. Rosenblat, *La población indígena*, 1:102.
89. Denevan, "Epilogue" (1976): 291.
90. Ibid. (1992): xxviii–xxix.
91. Kroeber, "Native American Population," 23–25.
92. Riccioli, *Geographiae Hydrographiae Reformatae*, 679–80.

93. Rivet and Loukotka, "Langues americaines," 597–712; Sapper, "Die Zahl und die Volksdichte der indianischen Bevolkerung in America," 1:95–104; and Spinden, "The Population of Ancient America," 641–61.

94. Willcox, "Increase of the Population of the Earth and of the Continents since 1650," 2:33–82.

95. Rosenblat, *La población indígena*, 1:102.

96. Borah, "America as Model: The Demographic Impact of European Expansion upon the Non-European World," 381.

97. Dobyns, "Estimating Aboriginal American Population," 414–15.

98. Morner, *Race Mixture in the History of Latin America*, 11–12.

99. Ubelaker, "Prehistoric New World Population Size," 661–65; Denevan, "Epilogue" (1976): 289–92; and Thornton, *American Indian Holocaust*, 22–25.

100. Denevan, "Native American Populations in 1492: Recent Research and a Revised Hemispheric Estimate" (1992): xvii–xxix.

101. Whitmore, *Disease and Death in Early Colonial Mexico*, 206–7; and Stannard, *American Indian Holocaust*, 262–68.

102. Cowley, "The Great Disease Migration," 54–56; and "America Before Columbus," 22–37.

103. Osborne, "The Numbers Game," 58.

Epilogue

1. Crosby, "Influenza," 810.

· Bibliography ·

Adams, Charles F. *Three Episodes in Massachusetts History*. Boston: Houghton, Mifflin and Company, 1903.

Alden, Dauril, and Joseph C. Miller. "Out of Africa: The Slave Trade and the Transmission of Smallpox to Brazil, 1560–1831." *Journal of Interdisciplinary History* 18 (1987): 195–224.

Allison, Marvin J. "Paleopathology in Peruvian and Chilean Populations." In *Paleopathology at the Origins of Agriculture*, eds. Mark N. Cohen and George J. Armelagos, pp. 515–29. New York: Academic Press, 1984.

"America Before Columbus." *US News & World Report*. 111 (July 8, 1991): 22–32.

Anderson, E. N. "Why Is Humoral Medicine So Popular?" *Social Science and Medicine* 25 (1987): 331–37.

Anghiera, Pietro Martire d'. *Décadas del Nuevo Mundo*. Mexico: J. Porrua, 1944.

Armelagos, George L. "Health and Disease in Prehistoric Populations in Transition." In *Diseases in Populations in Transition: Anthropological and Epidemiological Perspectives*. Edited by Alan C. Swedlund and George J. Armelagos, pp. 127–44. New York: Bergin & Garvey, 1990.

Arriaga, Pablo Jose de. *The Extirpation of Idolatry in Peru*. Translated and edited by L. Clark Keating. Lexington: University of Kentucky Press, 1968.

Astudillo Espinosa, Celín. *Páginas históricas de la medicina ecuatoriana: instituciones, ideas y personajes*. Quito: Instituto Panamericano de Geografía e Historia, 1981.

Austin Alchon, Suzanne. "Disease, Population and Public Health in Eighteenth-Century Quito." In *The Secret Judgments of God: Native Peoples and Old World Disease in Colonial Spanish America*. Edited by Noble David Cook and W. George Lovell, pp. 159–82. Norman: University of Oklahoma Press, 1992.

———. "The Great Killers in Precolumbian America: A Hemispheric Perspective." *The Latin American Population History Bulletin* 27 (1997), 2–10.

———. "Indians, Conquistadors, and Land in Early Sixteenth-Century Ecuador." Unpublished paper, 1998.

———. *Native Society and Disease in Colonial Ecuador*. New York: Cambridge University Press, 1991.

Bailey, Alfred G. *The Conflict of European and Eastern Algonkian Cultures, 1504–1700: A Study in Canadian Civilization.* Toronto: University of Toronto Press, 1969.

Bastien, Joseph W. *Healers of the Andes: Kallawaya Herbalists and Their Medicinal Plants.* Salt Lake City: University of Utah Press, 1987.

Begley, S., and A. Murr. "The First Americans." *Newsweek* 133:70 (April 26, 1999): 50–57.

Benedict, Carol. *Bubonic Plague in Nineteenth-Century China.* Stanford: Stanford University Press, 1996.

Betendorf, Joao Felipe. "Chronica da missao dos Padres da Companhia de Jesus," *Revista do Instituo Historico e Geographico Brasileiro* 22 (1901): 1-697.

Boccaccio, Giovanni. *The Decameron.* New York: W. W. Norton, 1982.

Bollet, Alfred Jay, and Audrey K. Brown. "Anemia." In *The Cambridge World History of Human Disease,* ed. Kenneth F. Kiple, pp. 571–77. New York: Cambridge University Press, 1993.

Borah, Woodrow. "America as Model: The Demographic Impact of European Expansion upon the Non-European World." *Actas y Memorias del XXXV Congreso Internacional de Americanistas.* Mexico, 3 (1964): 379–87.

Borah, Woodrow, and Sherburne F. Cook. *Essays in Population History: Mexico and the Caribbean.* 3 vols. Berkeley: University of California Press, 1971–1979.

Bourne, Edward G., ed. *Narratives of the Career of Hernando de Soto.* Translated by Buckingham Smith. New York: Allerton, 1922.

Boyd, Robert. "Commentary of Early Contact-Era Smallpox in the Pacific Northwest." *Ethnohistory* 43:2 (1996): 307–28.

———. "Population Decline from Two Epidemics on the Northwest Coast." In *Disease and Demography in the Americas,* eds. John Verano and Douglas Ubelaker, pp. 249–55. Washington: Smithsonian Institution Press, 1992.

Bradford, William. *History of Plymouth Plantation, 1620–1647.* Boston: The Massachusetts Historical Society, 1912.

Bratton, Timothy L. "The Identity of the New England Indian Epidemic of 1616–19." *Bulletin of the History of Medicine* 62:3 (1988): 351–83.

Brooks, Francis J. "Revising the Conquest of Mexico: Smallpox, Sources and Populations." *Journal of Interdisciplinary History* 24 (1993): 1–29.

Buikstra, Jane E. "Diseases of the Pre-Columbian Americas." In *The Cambridge World History of Human Disease.* Edited by Kenneth F. Kiple, pp. 305–17. New York: Cambridge University Press, 1993.

———. "Tuberculosis in the Americas: Current Perspectives." In *Human Paleopathology: Current Syntheses and Future Options.* Edited by Donald J. Ortner and Arthur C. Aufderheide, pp. 161–72. Washington, D.C.: Smithsonian Institution Press, 1991.

Burkholder, Mark, and Lyman Johnson. *Colonial Latin America.* New York: Oxford University Press, 1998.

Cabello de Balboa, Miguel. *Miscelanea antartica.* Lima: San Marcos, 1951.

Campbell, Sarah. *Post-Columbian Culture History in the Northern Columbia Plateau, A.D. 1500–1900.* New York: Garland Publishing, Inc., 1990.

Carlson, Catherine C., George J. Armelagos, and Ann L. Magennis. "Impact of Disease on Populations of New England and the Martimes." In *Disease and Demography in the Americas.* Edited by John Verano and Douglas Ubelaker, pp. 141–54. Washington, D.C.: Smithsonian Institution Press, 1992.

Carmichael, Ann G. "Leprosy." In *The Cambridge World History of Human Disease.* Edited by Kenneth F. Kiple, pp. 834–39. New York: Cambridge University Press, 1998.

———. *Plague and the Poor in Renaissance Florence.* New York: Cambridge University Press, 1986.

Carmichael, Ann G., and Arthur M. Silverstein. "Smallpox in Europe before the Seventeenth Century: Virulent Killer or Benign Disease?" In *Journal of the History of Medicine* 42 (1987): 147–68.

Cassidy, Claire M. "Skeletal Evidence for Prehistoric Subsistence Adaptation in the Central Ohio River Valley." In *Paleopathology at the Origins of Agriculture.* Edited by Mark N. Cohen and George L. Armelagos, pp. 307–45. New York: Academic Press, 1984.

Chakravorty, Ranes C. "Diseases of Antiquity in South Asia." In *The Cambridge World History of Human Disease.* Edited by Kenneth F. Kiple, pp. 408–12. New York: Cambridge University Press, 1993.

Chardon, Francis A. *Chardon's Journal at Fort Clark, 1834–1839.* Edited and with historical introduction and notes by Annie Heloise Abel. Lincoln: University of Nebraska Press, 1997.

Cieza de León, Pedro de. *The Discovery and Conquest of Peru: Chronicles of a New World Encounter.* Durham, N.C.: Duke University Press, 1998.

———. *Obras completas.* 3 vols. Madrid: Consejo Superior de Investigaciones Científicas, 1984–1985.

Cliff, Andrew D. *Measles: An Historical Geography of a Major Human Viral Disease from Global Expansion to Local Retreat, 1840–1990.* Cambridge, Mass.: Blackwell, 1993.

Cobo, Bernabé. *History of the Inca Empire: An Account of the Indians' Customs and their Origin, Together with a Treatise on Inca Legends, History, and Social Institutions.* Translated and edited by Roland Hamilton. Austin: University of Texas Press, 1979.

Cohen, Mark N., and George L. Armelagos, eds. *Paleopathology at the Origins of Agriculture.* New York: Academic Press, 1984.

Colección de documentos inéditos relativos al descubrimiento, conquista y organización de las antiguas posesiones españolas de America y Oceanía. Madrid: Academia de la Historia, 1964.

Cook, Della C. "Subsistence and Health in the Lower Illinois Valley: Osteological Evidence." In *Paleopathology at the Origins of Agriculture.* Edited by Mark N. Cohen and George L. Armelagos, pp. 237–70. New York: Academic Press, 1984.

Cook, Noble David. *Born to Die: Disease and New World Conquest, 1492–1650.* New York: Cambridge University Press, 1998.

———. *Demographic Collapse, Indian Peru, 1520–1620.* New York: Cambridge University Press, 1981.

———. "Disease and Depopulation of Hispaniola, 1492–1518." *Colonial Latin American Review* 2 (1993): 213–45.

———. "Impact of Disease in the Sixteenth-Century Andean World." In *Disease and Demography in the Americas.* Edited by John Verano and Douglas Ubelaker, pp. 207–13. Washington, D.C.: Smithsonian Institution Press, 1992.

Cook, Noble David, and W. George Lovell, eds. *The Secret Judgments of God: Native Peoples and Old World Disease in Colonial Spanish America.* Norman: University of Oklahoma Press, 1992.

Cook, Sherburne F. *The Conflict between the California Indian and White Civilization.* Berkeley: University of California Press, 1976.

———. "The Incidence and Significance of Disease Among the Aztecs and Related Tribes." *The Hispanic American Historical Review* 26 (1946): 320–35.

———. "The Significance of Disease in the Extinction of the New England Indian." *Human Biology* 45 (1973): 485–508.

Cook, Sherburne F., and Woodrow Borah. *The Aboriginal Population of Central Mexico on the Eve of the Spanish Conquest.* Berkeley: University of California Press, 1963.

———. "The Aboriginal Population of Hispaniola." In *Essays in Population History: Mexico and the Caribbean.* Edited by Sherburne F. Cook and Woodrow Borah, 1:376–410. Berkeley: University of California Press, 1971.

———. "Materials for the Demographic History of Mexico, 1500–1960." In *Essays in Population History: Mexico and the Caribbean.* Edited by Sherburne F. Cook and Woodrow Borah, 1:1–12. Berkeley: University of California Press, 1971.

Cook, Sherburne F., and Leslie B. Simpson. *The Population of Central Mexico in the Sixteenth Century.* Berkeley: University of California Press, 1948.

Cortés, Hernán. *Cartas de relación.* Mexico: Editorial Porrua, 1960.

———. *Letters from Mexico.* Translated and edited by A. R. Pagden. New York: Grossman Publishers, 1971.

Cowley, "The Great Disease Migration." *Newsweek,* Special Issue, (fall/winter 1991).

Crosby, Alfred W. "Conquistador y Pestilencia: The First New World Pandemic and the Fall of the Great Indian Empires." *Hispanic American Historical Review* 47 (1967): 321–37.

———. "Influenza." In *The Cambridge World History of Human Disease.* Edited by Kenneth F. Kiple, pp. 807–10. New York: Cambridge University Press, 1993.

———. "Summary on Population Size before and after Contact." In *Disease and Demography in the Americas.* Edited by John W. Verano and Douglas H. Ubelaker, pp. 277–78. Washington, D.C.: Smithsonian Institution Press, 1992.

Cybulski, Jerome S. "Culture Change, Demographic History, and Health and Disease on the Northwest Coast." In *In the Wake of Contact: Biological Responses to Conquest.* Edited by Clark S. Larsen and George R. Milner, pp. 75–86. New York: Wiley-Liss, 1994.

Dean, Warren. "Indigenous Populations of the São Paulo–Rio de Janeiro Coast: Trade, Aldeamento, Slavery and Extinction." *Revista Historica* (São Paulo) 117 (1984): 3–26.

Denevan, William M. *The Native Population of the Americas in 1492.* First edition, 1976, second edition 1992. Madison: University of Wisconsin Press.

Díaz del Castillo, Bernal. *The Conquest of Mexico.* New York: Viking Penguin, 1963.

Dixon, C. W. *Smallpox.* London: J. and A. Churchill, 1962.

Dobyns, Henry F. "Estimating Aboriginal American Population: An Appraisal of Techniques with a New Hemispheric Estimate." *Current Anthropology* 7 (1966): 395–449.

———. "An Outline of Andean Epidemic History to 1720." *Bulletin of the History of Medicine* 37 (1963): 493–515.

———. "Reassessing New World Populations at the Time of Contact." *Encuentro* 4:4 (1988): 8–9.

———. *Their Number Become Thinned: Native American Population Dynamics in Eastern North America.* Knoxville: University of Tennessee Press, 1983.

Dols, Michael. *Black Death in the Middle East.* Princeton, N.J.: Princeton University Press, 1977.

Driver, Harold E. *Indians of North America.* Chicago: University of Chicago Press, 1969.

Duffy, John. *Epidemics in Colonial America.* Baton Rouge: Louisiana State University Press, 1953.

Duncan, John D. "Indian Slavery." In *Race Relations in British North America, 1607–1783.* Edited by Bruce A. Glasrud and Alan M. Smith, pp. 85–106. Chicago: Nelson-Hall, 1982.

Duncan-Jones, R. P. "The Impact of the Antonine Plague." *Journal of Roman Archaeology* 9 (1996): 108–36.

Dunn, Frederick L. "Epidemiological Factors: Health and Disease in Hunter-Gatherers." In *Man the Hunter.* Edited by Richard B. Lee and Irven Defore, pp. 221–228. Chicago: Aldine Publishing Co., 1969.

Du Pratz, Le Page. *The History of Louisiana.* Baton Rouge: Louisiana State University Press, 1975.

Duran, Diego. *The History of the Indies of New Spain.* Translated by Doris Heyden. Norman: University of Oklahoma Press, 1994.

Estrada Ycaza, Julio. *El hospital de Guayaquil.* Guayaquil: Publicaciones del Archivo Historico del Guayas, 1973.

Farris, W. Wayne. "Diseases of the Premodern Period in Japan." In *The Cambridge World History of Human Disease.* Edited by Kenneth F. Kiple, pp. 376–84. New York: Cambridge University Press, 1993.

Federman, Nicolas. *Viaje a las Indias del Mar Oceano.* Buenos Aires: Editorial Nova, 1945.

Feldman, Lawrence. "Active Measures in the War Against Epidemics in Colonial Guatemala, 1519–1821." *Caduceus: A Museum Journal for the Health Sciences* 7, 3 (1991): 1–11.

Fenn, Elizabeth. "Biological Warfare Circa 1750." *The New York Times* (April 11, 1998), section A:25.

Fenner, F. *Smallpox and Its Eradication.* Geneva: World Health Association, 1988.

Fernandez del Castillo, Francisco. "El tifus en Mexico antes de Zinsser." In *Ensayos sobre la historia de las epidemias en Mexico.* Edited by Enrique Florescano and Elsa Malvido, 1:127–35. Mexico: Instituto de Seguro Social, 1982.

Fernandez de Oviedo y Valdez, Gonzalo. *Historia general y natural de las Indias, islas y tierrafirme de mar océano.* Madrid: Impresas de la Real Academia de la Historia, 1851.

Fieldhouse, D. K. *Colonial Empires: A Comparative Survey from the Eighteenth Century.* New York: Delacorte Press, 1967.

Figueroa Marroquin, Horacio. *Enfermedades de los conquistadors.* San Salvador: Ministerio de Cultura, Departmento Editorial, 1957.

Foster, George M. "On the Origin of Humoral Medicine in Latin America." *Medical Anthropology Quarterly* 1 (1987): 355–93.

Foucault, Michel. *Madness and Civilization; A History of Insanity in the Age of Reason.* Translated by Richard Howard. New York: Vintage Books, 1973.

Friede, Juan. "Demographic Changes in the Mining Community of Muzo After the Plague of 1629." *Hispanic American Historical Review* 47 (1967): 338–59.

Frost, Richard H. "The Pueblo Indian Smallpox Epidemic in New Mexico, 1898–1899." *Bulletin of the History of Medicine* 64 (1990): 417–45.

Fuentes y Guzman, Francisco Antonio de. *Recordación Florida.* Guatemala: Tipografia Nacional, 1933.

Gallagher, Nancy E. "Islamic and Indian Medicine." In *The Cambridge World History of Human Disease.* Edited by Kenneth F. Kiple, pp. 27–35. New York: Cambridge University Press, 1993.

Garcilaso de la Vega, El Inca. *The Florida of the Inca; A History of the Adelantado, Hernando de Soto, Governor and Captain General of the Kingdom of Florida, and of Other Heroic Spanish and Indian Cavaliers.* Translated and edited by John Grier Varner and Jeannette Johnson Varner. Austin: University of Texas Press, 1951.

———. *Royal Commentaries of the Incas, and General History of Peru.* 2 vols. Translated by Harold V. Livermore. Austin: University of Texas Press, 1966.

Garrett, Laurie. *The Coming Plague: Newly Emerging Diseases in a World Out of Balance.* New York: Farrar, Straus and Giroux, 1994.

Gerhard, Peter. *A Guide to the Historical Geography of New Spain.* Cambridge: Cambridge University Press, 1993.

Gerszten, Enrique, and M. J. Allison. "Human Soft Tissue Tumors in Paleopathology." In *Human Paleopathology: Current Synthesis and Future Options.* Edited by Donald J. Ortner and Arthur C. Aufderheide, pp. 257–60. Washington, D.C.: Smithsonian Institution Press, 1991.

Goodman, Alan H., John Lallo, George J. Armelagos, and Jerome C. Roe. "Health Changes at Dickson Mounds, Illinois (A.D. 950–1300). In *Paleopathology at the Origins of Agriculture.* Edited by Mark Cohen and George Armelagos, pp. 271–306. New York: Academic Press, 1984.

Gottfried, Robert. *The Black Death: Natural and Human Disaster in Medieval Europe.* London: Hale, 1983.

———. *Epidemic Disease in Fifteenth Century England: The Medical Response and the Demographic Consequences.* New Brunswick: Rutgers University Press, 1978.

Grmek, Mirko D. *Diseases in the Ancient Greek World.* Translated by Mireille Muellner and Leonard Muellner. Baltimore: The Johns Hopkins University Press, 1989.

Guaman Poma de Ayala, Felipe. *La nueva corónica y buen gobierno.* 3 vols. Lima: Editorial Cultura, 1956.

———. *Letter to a King: A Peruvian Chief's Account of Life under the Incas and under Spanish Rule.* Edited by Christopher Dilker. New York: E. P. Dutton, 1978.

Guerra, Francisco. "La epidemia americana de influenza en 1493." *Revista de Indias* 45 (1985): 325–47.

Gwei-Djen, Lu, and Joseph Needham. "Diseases of Antiquity in China." In *The Cambridge World History of Human Disease.* Edited by Kenneth F. Kiple, pp. 345–53. New York: Cambridge University Press, 1993.

Hann, John H. *Apalachee. The Land Between the Rivers.* Gainesville: University of Florida Press, 1988.

Hariot, Thomas. *A Briefe and True Report of the New Found Land of Virginia.* New York: History Book Club, 1951.

Harris, Cole. "Voices of Disaster: Smallpox Around the Strait of Georgia in 1782." *Ethnohistory* 41:4 (1994): 591–626.

Hemming, John. *Red Gold: The Conquest of the Brazilian Indians.* Cambridge, Mass.: Harvard University Press, 1978.

Henige, David. "Native American Population at Contact." *Latin American Population History Bulletin* 22 (1992): 2–23.

———. *Numbers from Nowhere: The American Indian Contact Population Debate.* Norman: University of Oklahoma Press, 1998.

———. "On the Contact Population of Hispaniola: History as Higher Mathematics." *Hispanic American Historical Review* 58 (1978): 217–37.

Herlihy, David. *The Black Death and the Transformation of the West.* Cambridge, Mass.: Harvard University Press, 1997.

———. "The Bright Side of the Plague." *The New York Review* (March 4, 1999): 26–28.

Hernández, Francisco. *Obras completas.* 6 vols. Mexico: UNAM, 1959–1985.

Hernández Rodríguez, Rosaura. "Epidemias y calamides en el Mexico prehispanico." In *Ensayos sobre la historia de las epidemias en Mexico.* Edited by Enrique Florescano and Elsa Malvido, 1:215–31. Mexico: Instituto Mexicano del Seguro Social, 1982.

Herrera y Tordesillas, Antonio de. *Historia general de los hechos de los castellanos en las islas y tierra firme del Mar Océano.* 17 vols. Madrid: Real Academia de la Historia, 1934.

Hopkins, Donald. *Princes and Peasants: Smallpox in History.* Chicago: University of Chicago Press, 1983.

Hughes, Donald J. *American Indian Ecology.* El Paso: Texas Western Press, 1983.

Jaffee, A. J. *The First Immigrants from Asia.* New York: Plenum Press, 1992.

Jantz, Richard L., and Douglas W. Owsley. "White Traders in the Upper Missouri: Evidence from the Swan Creek Site." In *Skeletal Biology in the Great Plains: Migration, Warfare, Health and Subsistence.* Edited by Douglas W. Owsley and Richard L. Jantz, pp. 189–202. Washington, D.C.: Smithsonian Institution Press, 1994.

Jimenez de la Espada, Marcos, ed. *Relaciones geográficas de Indias: Peru.* 3 vols. Madrid: Atlas, 1965.

Johnson, H. B. "Portuguese Settlement, 1500–1580." In *Colonial Brazil.* Edited by Leslie Bethell, pp. 1–38. Cambridge: Cambridge University Press, 1987.

Kilbourne, Edwin D. *Influenza.* New York: Plenum Publishing Co., 1987.

Kiple, Kenneth F. "Diseases of Sub-Saharan Africa to 1860." In *The Cambridge World History of Human Disease.* Edited by Kenneth F. Kiple, pp. 293–97. New York: Cambridge University Press, 1993.

———. "Skeletal Biology and the History of Native Americans and African Americans." In *The Latin American Population History Bulletin* 21 (1992): 3–10.

Kroeber, A. L. "Native American Population." *American Anthropologist* 36:1 (1934): 1–25.

Landa, Diego de. *Landa's Relación de las Cosas de Yucatán, a Translation.* Cambridge, Mass.: The Museum, 1941.

Larsen, Clarke. "Health and Disease in Prehistoric Georgia." In *Paleopathology at the Origins of Agriculture.* Edited by Mark N. Cohen and George L. Armelagos, pp. 367–392. New York: Academic Press, 1984.

———. "In the Wake of Columbus: Native Population Biology in the Postcontact Americas." In *The Yearbook of Physical Anthropology* 37 (1994): 115–25.

Larsen, Clarke, Christopher Ruff, Margaret Schoeninger, and Dale Hutchinson. "Population Decline and Extinction in La Florida." In *Disease and Demography in the Americas.* Edited by John Verano and Douglas Ubelaker, pp. 25–40. Washington, D.C.: Smithsonian Institution Press, 1992.

Las Casas, Bartolomé de. *Historia de las Indias.* 3 vols. Mexico: Fondo de Cultura Economica, 1951.

———. *A Short Account of the Destruction of the Indies.* Edited and Translated by Nigel Griffin. London: Penguin Books, 1992.

León, Nicholas. "Que era el Matlazahuatl y que el Cocoliztli en los tiempos precolumbinos y en la epoca hispana?" In *Ensayos sobre la historia de las epidemias en Mexico.* Edited by Enrique Florescano and Elsa Malvido, 1:385–411. Mexico: Instituto del Seguro Social, 1982.

Lery, Jean de. *History of a Voyage to the Land of Brazil, Otherwise Called America.* Translated by Janet Whatley. Berkeley: University of California Press, 1990.

Levillier, Roberto. *Gobernantes del Perú, cartas y papeles, siglo XVI; documentos del Archivo de Indias*. Madrid: Sucesores de Rivadeneyra, 1925.

Lopez Austin, Alfredo. *The Human Body and Ideology: Concepts of the Ancient Nahuas*. Salt Lake City: University of Utah Press, 1988.

López de Gómara, Francisco. *Cortés: The Life of the Conqueror by His Secretary*. Translated and edited by Lesley Byrd Simpson. Berkeley: University of California Press, 1964.

Lovell, W. George. *Conquest and Survival in Colonial Guatemala: A Historical Geography of the Cuchumatán Highlands*. Kingston: McGill-Queen's University Press, 1985.

———. "Disease in Early Colonial Guatemala." In *Secret Judgments of God: Old World Disease in Colonial Spanish America*. Edited by Noble David Cook and W. George Lovell, pp. 49–83. Norman: University of Oklahoma Press, 1992.

Lovell, W. George, and Christopher H. Lutz. *Demography and Empire: A Guide to the Population History of Spanish Central America, 1500–1821*. Boulder, Colo.: Westview Press, 1995.

MacLeod, Murdo J. *Spanish Central America: A Socioeconomic History, 1520–1720*. Berkeley: University of California Press, 1973.

MacLeod, William C. *The American Indian Frontier*. New York: Alfred A. Knopf, 1928.

Malvido, Elsa. "Cronología de epidemias." In *Ensayos sobre la historia de las epidemias en Mexico*. Edited by Enrique Florescano and Elsa Malvido, pp. 171–76. Mexico: Instituto de Seguro Social, 1982.

Martinez, Duran. *Las ciencias médicas en Guatemala, origen y evolución*. Guatemala: Tipografia Sanchez y De Guise, 1941.

McBryde, Felix W. "Influenza in America during the Sixteenth Century (Guatemala: 1523, 1559–1562, 1576)." *Bulletin of the History of Medicine* 8 (1940): 296–302.

McCaa, Robert. "Paradise, Hells, and Purgatories: Population, Health, and Nutrition in Mexican History and Prehistory." Unpublished paper, 1993.

———. "Spanish and Nahuatl Views on Smallpox and Demographic Catastrophe in Mexico." *Journal of Interdisciplinary History* 25:3 (1995): 397–431.

McGrath, J. W. "A Computer Simulation of the Spread of Tuberculosis in Prehistoric Populations of the Lower Illinois River Valley." Ph.D. dissertation, Northwestern University, 1986.

McNeill, William H. *Plagues and Peoples*. Garden City, N.Y.: Anchor Books, 1976.

Merbs, Charles F. "A New World of Infectious Disease." *Yearbook of Physical Anthropology* 35:3 (1992): 3–42.

Milanich, Jerald T. *Florida Indians and the Invasion from Europe*. Gainesville: University of Florida Press, 1995.

Miller, J. R. *Skyscrapers Hide the Heavens: A History of Indian-White Relations in Canada*. Toronto: University of Toronto Press, 2000.

Miller, Judith, Stephen Engleberg, and William Broad. *Germs: Biological Weapons and America's Secret War*. New York: Simon and Schuster, 2001.

Milner, George. "Disease and Sociopolitical Systems in Late Prehistoric Illinois." In *Disease and Demography in the Americas*. Edited by John Verano and Douglas Ubelaker, pp. 103–16. Washington, D.C.: Smithsonian Institution Press, 1992.

———. "Epidemic Disease in the Postcontact Southeast: A Reappraisal." *Midcontinental Journal of Archaeology* 5 (1980): 39–56.

Mooney, James. *The Aboriginal Population of America North of Mexico*. Washington, D.C.: Smithsonian Institution, 1928.

Moore, R. I. *The Formation of a Persecuting Society: Power and Deviance in Western Europe, 950–1250*. New York: B. Blackwell, 1987.

Morner, Magnus. *Race Mixture in the History of Latin America*. Boston: Little, Brown and Co., 1967.

Motolinia o Benavente, Toribio de. *Memoriales; o libro de las cosas de la Nueva España y de los naturales de ella*. Mexico: UNAM, 1971.

Moya Pons, Frank. *Después de Colón: trabajo, sociedad y política en la economía del oro*. Madrid: Alianza, 1987.

———. *La Española en el siglo XVI, 1493–1520*. Santiago de los Caballeros: UCMM, 1971.

Nabokov, Peter. *Native American Testimony: A Chronicle of Indian-White Relations from Prophecy to the Present*. New York: Penguin, 1991.

Nasatir, A. P. *Before Lewis and Clark: Documents Illustrating the History of the Missouri, 1785–1804*. St. Louis: St. Louis Historical Documents Foundation, 1952.

Nester, William R. *The Great Frontier War: Britain, France and the Imperial Struggle for North America*. Westport, Conn.: Praeger, 2000.

Newman, "Aboriginal New World Epidemiology and Medical Care, and the Impact of Old World Disease Imports." *American Journal of Physical Anthropology* 45 (1976): 667–72.

Newson, Linda. *The Cost of Conquest: Indian Decline in Honduras Under Spanish Rule*. Boulder, Colo.: Westview Press, 1986.

———. "The Depopulation of Nicaragua in the Sixteenth Century." *Journal of Latin American Studies* 14 (1982): 253–86.

———. *Indian Survival in Colonial Nicaragua*. Norman: University of Oklahoma Press, 1987.

———. *Life and Death in Early Colonial Ecuador*. Norman: University of Oklahoma Press, 1995.

———. "Old World Epidemics in Early Colonial Ecuador." In *Secret Judgments of God: Old World Disease in Colonial Spanish America*. Edited by Noble David Cook and W. George Lovell, pp. 84–112. Norman: University of Oklahoma Press, 1992.

Oberg, Michael L. *Dominion and Civility: English Imperialism and Native America, 1585–1685*. Ithaca, N.Y.: Cornell University Press, 1999.

O'Neill, Ynez Viole. "Diseases of the Middle Ages." In *The Cambridge World History of Human Disease*. Edited by Kenneth F. Kiple, pp. 270–78. New York: Cambridge University Press, 1993.

Orellana, Sandra L. *Indian Medicine in Highland Guatemala: The Pre-Hispanic and Colonial Periods*. Albuquerque: University of New Mexico Press, 1987.

Ortiz de Montellano, Bernard. *Aztec Medicine, Health, and Nutrition*. New Brunswick, N.J.: Rutgers University Press, 1990.

Ortner, Donald J. "Diseases of the Pre-Roman World." In *The Cambridge World History of Human Disease*. Edited by Kenneth F. Kiple, pp. 247–61. New York: Cambridge University Press, 1993.

———. "Skeletal Paleopathology." In *Disease and Demography in the Americas*. Edited by John W. Verano and Douglas H. Ubelaker, pp. 5–14. Washington, D.C.: Smithsonian Institution Press, 1992.

Osborne, Lawrence. "The Numbers Game: Can Historians Count?" *Lingua Franca* (September 1998): 50–58.

Owsley, Douglas. "Demography of Prehistoric and Early Historic Northern Plains Populations." In *Disease and Demography in the Americas*. Edited by John Verano and Douglas Ubelaker, pp. 75–86. Washington, D.C.: Smithsonian Institution Press, 1992.

Pagden, Anthony. *Lords of All the World: Ideologies of Empire in Spain, Britain and France, c. 1500–c. 1800.* New Haven, Conn.: Yale University Press, 1995.

Paredes Borja, Virgilio. *Historia de la medicina en el Ecuador.* 2 vols. Quito: Editorial Casa de la Cultura Ecuatoriana, 1963.

Park, Katharine. "Black Death." In *The Cambridge World History of Human Disease.* Edited by Kenneth F. Kiple, pp. 612–16. New York: Cambridge University Press, 1993.

Paso y Troncoso, Francisco del. *Epistolario de Nueva España, 1505–1818.* Mexico: Antigua librería Robredo, 1940.

Patterson, K. David. *Pandemic Influenza, 1700–1900.* Totowa, N.J.: Rowman and Littlefield, Publishers, 1986.

Phelan, John L. *The Kingdom of Quito in the Seventeenth Century; Bureaucratic Politics in the Spanish Empire.* Madison: University of Wisconsin Press, 1967.

Porras Barrenecha, Raul. *Cartas del Perú, 1524–1543.* Lima: Sociedad de Bibliófilos Peruanos, 1959.

Powers, Karen V. *Andean Journeys: Migration, Ethnogenesis, and the State in Colonial Quito.* Albuquerque: University of New Mexico Press, 1995.

Prem, Hanns J. "Disease Outbreaks in Central Mexico during the Sixteenth Century." In *Secret Judgments of God: Old World Disease in Colonial Spanish America.* Edited by Noble David Cook and W. George Lovell, pp. 20–48. Norman: University of Oklahoma Press, 1992.

Ramenofsky, Ann F. *Vectors of Death: The Archaeology of European Contact.* Albuquerque: University of New Mexico Press, 1987.

Recinos, Adrian, and Delia Goetz, eds. *Annals of the Cakchiquels.* Norman: University of Oklahoma Press, 1953.

Reff, Daniel. *Disease, Depopulation, and Culture Change in Northwestern New Spain, 1518–1764.* Salt Lake City: University of Utah Press, 1991.

Reinhard, Karl J., et al. "Trade, Contact, and Female Health in Northeast Nebraska." In *In the Wake of Contact: Biological Responses to Conquest.* Edited by Clark S. Larsen and George L. Milner, pp. 63–74. New York: Wiley-Liss, 1994.

Riccioli, Giovanni Battista. *Geographiae Hydrographiae Reformatae nuper recognitae el auctae libri duodecimi.* Venice: Typus I. La Nou, 1672.

Risse, Guenter B. "History of Western Medicine from Hippocrates to Germ Theory." In *The Cambridge World History of Human Disease.* Edited by Kenneth F. Kiple, pp. 11–19. New York: Cambridge University Press, 1993.

Rivet, Paul, G. Stresser-Pean, and C. Loukotka. "Langues americaines." In *Les langues du monde.* Edited by A. Meillet and M. Cohen, 16:597–712. Paris: Société de Linguistique de Paris, 1924.

Rodriguez Demorizi, Emilio. *Los domínicos y las encomiendas de indios de la isla Española.* Santo Domingo: Editorial del Caribe, 1971.

Rosenblat, Angel. "El desarrollo de la población indígena de America." *Tierra Firme* 1:1 (1935): 115–33; 1:2 (1935); 117–48; 1:3 (1935): 109–41.

———. *La población indígena y el mestizaje en América.* 2 vols. Buenos Aires: Editorial Nova, Biblioteca Americanista, 1954.

———. "The Population of Hispaniola at the Time of Columbus." In *The Native Population of the Americas in 1492.* Edited by William M. Denevan, pp. 43–66. Madison: University of Wisconsin Press, 1992.

Royal, Robert. *Columbus on Trial: 1492 v. 1992.* Herndon, VA: Young Americas Foundation, 1992.

Rowe, John H. "Inca Culture at the Time of the Spanish Conquest." In *Handbook of South American Indians.* Edited by Julian H. Steward. 2 (1946): 183–330.

Roys, Ralph L. *The Book of Chilam Balam of Chumayel.* Norman: University of Oklahoma Press, 1967.

Ruiz de Alarcón, Hernando. *Treatise on the Heathen Superstitions that Today Live among the Indians Native to This New Spain, 1629.* Translated and Edited by J. Richard Andrews and Ross Hassig. Norman: University of Oklahoma Press, 1984.

Russell, Josiah C. *Late Ancient and Medieval Population.* Philadelphia: American Philosophical Society, 1958.

Sahagún, Bernardino de. *Florentine Codex: General History of the Things of New Spain.* Edited by Arthur O. Anderson and Charles E. Dibble. 13 vols. Santa Fe, N.Mex.: School of American Research, 1950–1982.

———. *Historia general de las cosas de Nueva España.* Mexico: Editorial Porrua, 1992.

Said, Mohammed. "Diseases of the Premodern Period in South Asia." In *The Cambridge World History of Human Disease.* Edited by Kenneth F. Kiple, pp. 413–17. New York: Cambridge University Press, 1993.

Sale, Kirkpatrick. *The Conquest of Paradise: Christopher Columbus and the Columbian Legacy.* New York: Alfred A. Knopf, 1990.

Salomon, Frank and George L. Urioste, trans. *The Huarochiri Manuscript: A Testament of Ancient and Colonial Andean Religion.* Austin: University of Texas Press, 1991.

Sancho Paz Ponce de Leon, Juan. "Relacion y descripcion de los pueblos del partido de Otavalo." In *Relaciones geograficas de Indias.* 3 vols. Edited by Marcos Jimenez de la Espada, 3: 233–40. Madrid: Atlas, 1965.

Sanders, William. *The Teotihuacan Valley Project.* University Park: Occasional Papers in Anthropology, Pennsylvania State University, 1970.

Santa Cruz Pachacuti Yamqui Salcamayhua, Juan de. *Relación de antigüedades deste reyno del Piru.* Cusco: Centro de Estudios Regionales Andinos Bartolome de las Casas, 1993.

Sapper, Karl. "Die Zahl und die Volksdichte der indianischen Bevolkerung in America vor der Conquista und der Gegenwart." In Proceedings of the 21st International Congress of Americanists. 1 (1924): 95–104.

Sarmiento de Gamboa, Pedro. *Historia de los Incas.* Madrid: Miraguano Ediciones, 2001.

Saunders, Shelley, Peter Ramsden, and D. Ann Herring. "Transformation and Disease: Precontact Ontario Iroquoians." In *Disease and Demography in the Americas.* Edited by John W. Verano and Douglas H. Ubelaker, pp. 117–26. Washington, D.C.: Smithsonian Institution Press, 1992.

Seaver, Kirsten A. *The Frozen Echo: Greenland and the Exploration of North America, ca. A.D. 1000–1500.* Stanford: Stanford University Press, 1996.

Seed, Patricia. *Ceremonies of Possession in Europe's Conquest of the New World, 1492–1640.* New York: Cambridge University Press, 1995.

Shea, Daniel E. "A Defense of Small Population Estimates for the Central Andes in 1520." In *The Native Population of the Americas in 1492.* Edited by William M. Denevan, pp. 157–80. Madison: University of Wisconsin Press, 1976.

Sherman, William L. *Forced Native Labor in Sixteenth-Century Central America.* Lincoln: University of Nebraska Press, 1979.

Shigehisa, Kuriyama. "Concepts of Disease in East Asia." In *The Cambridge World History of Human Disease.* Edited by Kenneth F. Kiple, pp. 52–59. New York: Cambridge University Press, 1993.

Sleeper-Smith, Susan. "Women, Kin and Catholicism: New Perspectives on the Fur Trade." *Ethnohistory* 47:2 (2000): 423–52.

Slicher von Bath, B. H. "The Calculation of the Population of New Spain, Especially for the Period before 1570." *Boletin de estudios Latinoamericanos y del Caribe* 24 (1978): 67–95.

Smith, Craig S. "Virus Spreading by Ducks Spurs Immunologists." *The Wall Street Journal,* April 25, 1995. Section B:1.

Smith, C. T. "Depopulation of the Central Andes in the 16th Century." *Current Anthropology* 11: 4 (1970): 453–64.

Snow, D. R., and K. M. Lamphear. "European Contact and Indian Depopulation in the Northeast: The Timing of the First Epidemics." *Ethnohistory* 35 (1987): 15–33.

Spalding, Karen. *Huarochirí, An Andean Society Under Inca and Spanish Rule.* Stanford: Stanford University Press, 1984.

Spence, Lewis. *Myths and Legends of the North American Indians.* Blauvelt, N.Y.: Multimedia Publishing Corp., 1975.

Spinden, Herbert J. "The Population of Ancient America." *The Geographical Review* 18 (1928): 641–60.

Staden, Hans. *Hans Staden: The True Story of His Captivity, 1557.* London: Routledge and Sons, Ltd., 1928.

Stannard, David E. *American Indian Holocaust: Columbus and the Conquest of the New World.* New York: Oxford University Press, 1992.

Stannard, Jerry. "Diseases of Western Antiquity." In *The Cambridge World History of Human Disease.* Edited by Kenneth F. Kiple, pp. 262–69. New York: Cambridge University Press, 1993.

St Cosme, J. F. B. "Letter to the Bishop of Quebec." In *Early Voyages Up and Down the Mississippi.* Edited by L. C. Shea. Albany: Joel Munsell, 1861.

Stearn, Esther W., and Allen E. Stearn. *The Effect of Smallpox on the Destiny of the American Indian.* Boston: Bruce Humphries, 1945.

Stengel, M. F. "The Diffusionists Have Landed." *Atlantic Monthly* 285:1 (January 2000): 35–39.

Stern, Steve J. *Peru's Indian Peoples and the Challenge of Spanish Conquest: Huamanga to 1640.* Madison: University of Wisconsin Press, 1982.

Steward, Julian H. "The Native Population of South America." In *Handbook of South American Indians.* Edited by Julian H. Steward. 5 (1949): 655–68.

Stiffarm, Lenore A., and Phil Lane, Jr. "The Demography of Native North America: A Question of American Indian Survival." In *The State of Native America: Genocide, Colonization, and Resistance.* Edited by M. Annette Jaimes, pp. 23–54. Boston: South Press, 1992.

Stodder, Ann, and Debra Martin. "Health and Disease in the Southwest Before and After Spanish Contact." In *Disease and Demography in the Americas.* Edited by John Verano and Douglas Ubelaker, pp. 55–74. Washington, D.C.: Smithsonian Institution Press, 1992.

Storey, Rebecca. *Life and Death in the Ancient City of Teotihuacan: A Modern Paleodemographic Synthesis.* Tuscaloosa: University of Alabama Press, 1992.

Sundstrom, Linea. "Smallpox Used Them Up: References to Epidemic Disease in Northern Plains Winter Counts." *Ethnohistory* 44:2 (1997): 305–43.

Tello, Fray Antonio. *Libro segundo de la Crónica Miscelánea de la Santa Provincia de Xalisco.* Guadalajara: La República Literaria, 1891.

Thornton, Russell. *American Indian Holocaust and Survival: A Population History since 1492.* Norman: University of Oklahoma Press, 1987.

———. *We Shall Live Again: The 1870 and 1890 Ghost Dance Movements as Demographic Revitalization.* New York: Cambridge University Press, 1986.

Thucydides. *The Landmark: A Comprehensive Guide to the Peloponnesian War.* New York: Free Press, 1996.

Thwaites, Reuben G. *Jesuit Relations and Allied Documents*. Cleveland: Burrows Bros., 1896.

Toribio Polo, Jose. "Apuntes sobre las epidemias del Peru." *Revista historica* 5 (1913): 50–109.

Trimble, Michael K. "The 1837–38 Smallpox Epidemic on the Upper Missouri." In *Skeletal Biology in the Great Plains: Migration, Warfare, Health and Subsistence.* Edited by Douglas W. Owsley and Richard L. Jantz, pp. 81–90. Washington, D.C.: Smithsonian Institution Press, 1994.

Truteau, Zenon. "Journal of Truteau on the Missouri River, 1794–1795." In *Before Lewis and Clark: Documents Illustrating the History of the Missouri, 1785–1804.* Edited by A. P. Nasatir, pp. 259–311. St. Louis: St. Louis Historical Documents Foundation, 1952.

Tyrer, Robson B. "The Demographic and Economic History of the Audiencia of Quito: The Indian Population and the Textile Industry, 1600–1800." Ph.D. dissertation, Department of History, University of California, 1976.

Ubelaker, Douglas. "North American Indian Population Size, A.D. 1500–1985." *American Journal of Physical Anthropology* 77:3 (1988): 289–94.

———. "Prehistoric New World Population Size: Historical Review and Current Appraisal of North American Estimates." *American Journal of Physical Anthropology* 45 (1976): 661–66.

———. "The Sources and Methodology for Mooney's Estimates of North American Indian Populations." In *The Native Population of the Americas in 1492.* Edited by William M. Denevan, pp. 243–88. Madison: University of Wisconsin Press, 1992.

Unschuld, Paul U. "History of Chinese Medicine." In *The Cambridge World History of Human Disease.* Edited by Kenneth F. Kiple, pp. 20–27. New York: Cambridge University Press, 1993.

Veblen, Thomas T. "Native Population Decline in Totonicapan, Guatemala." *Annals of the Association of American Geographers* 67 (1977): 484–99.

Verano, John W. "Prehistoric Disease and Demography in the Andes." In *Disease and Demography in the Americas.* Edited by John W. Verano and Douglas H. Ubelaker, pp. 15–24. Washington, D.C.: Smithsonian Institution Press, 1992.

Verlinden, Charles. "La population de l'Amerique précolumbienne: une question de méthode." In *Méthodologie de l'histoire et des sciences humaines: mélanges en honneur de Fernand Braudel,* pp. 453–62. Paris: 1973.

Vibert, Elizabeth. "The Natives Were Strong to Live: Reinterpreting Early-Nineteenth-Century Prophetic Movements in the Columbia Plateau." *Ethnohistory* 42:2 (1995): 197–229.

Villamarin, Juan and Judith. "Epidemic Disease in the Sabana de Bogota." In *Secret Judgments of God: Old World Disease in Colonial Spanish America.* Edited by Noble David Cook and W. George Lovell, pp. 113–41. Norman: University of Oklahoma Press, 1992.

———. *Indian Labor in Mainland Colonial Spanish America.* Newark: University of Delaware, Latin American Studies Program, 1975.

Virrey Conde del Villar, "Virrey Conde del Villar a los médicos y oficiales del Virreinato del Peru, Lima, March 21, 1589." Latin American Manuscripts Collection, Peru Manuscripts Department, Lilly Library, Indiana University, Bloomington.

Wachtel, Nathan. *The Vision of the Vanquished: The Spanish Conquest of Peru through Indian Eyes, 1530–1570.* New York: Barnes and Noble, 1977.

Walker, Phillip, and John Johnson. "The Decline of the Chumash Indian Population." In *In the Wake of Contact: Biological Responses to Conquest.* Edited by Clark S. Larsen and George R. Milner, pp. 109–20. New York: Wiley-Liss, 1994.

———. "Effects of Contact on the Chumash Indians." In *Disease and Demography in the Americas*. Edited by John Verano and Douglas Ubelaker, pp. 127–40. Washington, D.C.: Smithsonian Institution Press, 1992.

Walker, Phillip, P. Lambert, and M. DeNiro. "The Effects of European Contact on the Health of California Indians." In *Columbian Consequences*, vol. 1: *Archaeological and Historical Perspective on the Spanish Borderlands West*. Edited by David H. Thomas, pp. 349–64. Washington, D.C.: Smithsonian Institution, 1989.

Watts, Sheldon. *Epidemics in History: Disease, Power and Imperialism*. New Haven, Conn.: Yale University Press, 1997.

Weiss, Rick. "Bioterrorism: An Ever More Devastating Threat." *The Washington Post*. September 17, 2001, Section A, p. A24.

Whitmore, Thomas M. *Disease and Death in Early Colonial Mexico: Simulating Amerindian Population Decline*. Boulder: University of Colorado Press, 1992.

———. "A Simulation of the Sixteenth-Century Population Collapse in the Basin of Mexico." *Annals of the Association of American Geographers* 81 (1991): 464–87.

Willcox, Walter. "Increase of the Population of the Earth and of the Continents since 1650. In *International Migrations*. Edited by Walter Willcox, pp. 33–82. New York: National Bureau of Economic Research, 1931.

Wood, Peter H. "The Changing Population of the Colonial South: An Overview by Race and Region, 1685–1790." In *Powhatan's Mantle: Indians in the Colonial Southeast*. Edited by Peter H. Wood, Gregory A. Waselkov, and M. Thomas Hartley, pp. 35–103. Lincoln: University of Nebraska Press, 1989.

Zambardino, Rudolph A. "A Critique of David Henige's 'On the Contact Population of Hispaniola': History as Higher Mathematics." *Hispanic American Historical Review* 58 (1978): 700–708.

———. "Errors in Historical Demography." *The Institute of Mathematics and Its Applications* 17 (1981): 238–40.

———. "Review of Noble David Cook, *Demographic Collapse*."

———. "Review of *Demographic Collapse: Indian Peru, 1520–1620*." *Journal of Interdisciplinary History* 14 (1984): 719–22.

Zinsser, Hans. *Rats, Lice and History*. Boston: Little, Brown and Co., 1941.

• Index •

Note: The notations *f* and *t* indicate figures and tables on the respective pages.

Missouri, 104
mita, 140
Mixton War, 126
modorra, 62–63, 91
Mongol Empire, 28
morbidity rates, 81
mortality rates, Andean region, 77–78;
    Brazil, 86; Brazil and North America
    compared, 106; California, 100;
    Central America, 71; Florida, 93;
    Great Plains, 105; Guatemala, 75;
    Hispaniola, 64; Honduras, 74–75;
    Hopi, 123; hunter-gatherers, 39–45;
    infant and child, 39; infants and
    children, 44–45; Mexico, 66, 69–70;
    modern times, 80; New England, 98;
    Nicaragua, 74–75; northeastern U.S.,
    99; Old World before 1500, 21t,
    31; Pacific Northwest, 102–3;
    pre-Columbian, 42; regional varia-
    tions, 81; skeletal remains, 38;
    Teotihuacan, 38; twentieth century,
    108; typhus, 55; virgin soil epi-
    demics, 9, 80, 106
mumps, Mexico, 70
Muskogean speakers, 47

Na-Dene speakers, 46
Natchez peoples, 114
native Americans, arrival in New
    World, 33–34; common ancestry,
    34; conflicting beliefs, 112; creation
    myths, 32; explaining disease,
    110–11; pre-Columbian health,
    36–39; religious causation, 11;
    response, 116; romanticizing, 2–3;
    stereotyping, 3
Nayarit, 94
New England, 84, 96; first epidemic, 97,
    122; nursing care, 123
New France, 84, 96, 130–31
New Mexico, 94–95
New Spain. See Mexica; Mexico
New World, population estimates,
    170–72, 171f; regions of Americas
    (map), 35; simultaneous arrival of
    disease, 81–82, 143
New World leishmaniasis, 44
New World spotted fever, 44
Nicaragua, 73t, 74, 137
nomadic peoples, 42, 44
North Africa, 16
North America, 90–91; Brazil compared,
    105–8; early account, 90–91;
    European colonization, 83–84;
    Florida and the Southeast, 91–94;
    inoculation, 122; nadir population,
    159; population, 153–54, 156–60,
    158f; quarantines, 120; smallpox, 83;
    typhus, 56

North Carolina, 94
North Dakota, 103–4
northeastern U.S., 97t, 97–99
northern Mexico, 94–95, 95t
Norway, 90
Nova Scotia, 96–97
nursing care, 123

Old World, 4; dying patient as conta-
    gious, 14f; epidemics, frequency of,
    30–31; health-care practitioners, 10f;
    life expectancies, 53; mortality rates,
    82; New World compared, 3–4; phar-
    macist, 12f; regions, disease pattern
    map, 8; single pathogen, 143
origins and history of human disease,
    early, 15–18
Ottawa, 99

Pacific Islanders, 7, 34
Pacific Northwest, 45–46, 100–103, 107,
    115–16, 117
Paleo-Eskimo, 90
Pamunkey people, 134
Panama, 48, 67, 73t, 74
pandemics, 7, 29, 174
Paraguay, 88
parasitic infections, 43; Africa, 19; India,
    19; iron losses, 52; Middle East, 17;
    pre-Columbian, 53
paratyphoid fevers, 17
Patagonia, 40–41
patterns of disease, civilization-specific,
    16–17; history, studying, 17
pellagra, 52
Peloponnesian War, 24, 81
Penutian languages, 46
Peru, 75–76; abuse of natives, 136f;
    attacks on native communities,
    106; creation myths, 32; population,
    151–52, 154; quarantine, 120; small-
    pox, 114; violence, 126
Philippines, 22
pinta, 44, 54
pinworms, 43
plague, Brazil, 87; England, 28; France,
    28; Germany, 28; Italy, 28; Northern
    New Spain, 95t, 95; southern Spain,
    62; Spain, 28; tropical conditions, 75
Plague of Antonius, 25
Plague of Justinian, 28; mortality rates,
    31; smallpox, 31
Pleistocene, 33
pleurisy, New France, 97
pneumonia, 43; California, 100; China,
    20; Europe, 23; Hispaniola, 64;
    hunter-gatherers, 44; India, 19; non-
    immune individuals, 16; temperate
    North America, 56
pneumonic plague, 71, 76t, 76, 176